MW00720270

$ 7.00

PANDEMIC

PANDEMIC

THE TERRIFYING THREAT OF THE NEW KILLER PLAGUES

Pete Moore, Ph.D.

CITADEL PRESS
Kensington Publishing Corporation
kensingtonbooks.com

CITADEL PRESS BOOKS are published by

Kensington Publishing Corp.
850 Third Avenue
New York, NY 10022

Copyright © 2001 Pete Moore

All rights reserved. No part of this book may be reproduced in any form or by any means without the prior written consent of the publisher, excepting brief quotes used in reviews.

This is an unaltered reprint of the hardcover edition published in the United Kingdom under the title *Superbugs: Rogue Diseases of the Twenty-first Century* by Carlton Books Limited.

All Kensington titles, imprints, and distributed lines are available at special quantity discounts for bulk purchases for sales promotions, premiums, fund-raising, educational, or institutional use. Special book excerpts or customized printings can also be created to fit specific needs. For details, write or phone the office of the Kensington special sales manager: Kensington Publishing Corp., 850 Third Avenue, New York, NY 10022, attn: Special Sales Department; phone 1-800-221-2647.

CITADEL PRESS and the Citadel logo are Reg. U.S. Pat. & TM Off.

First printing: April 2007

10 9 8 7 6 5 4 3 2 1

Printed in the United States of America

Library of Congress Control Number: 2006935126

ISBN-13: 978-0-8065-2818-2
ISBN-10: 0-8065-2818-4

CONTENTS

PANDEMIC

CHAPTER 1 –
CONTEMPORARY COMPLACENCY

"We stand on the brink of a global crisis in infectious diseases. No country is safe from them. No country can any longer afford to ignore their threat," said Gro Harlem Brundtland while she held the post of Director-General of the World Health Organisation.[1] Surely she was getting emotional. She must have got so wrapped up in her job and have been spending so much time thinking about ill people that she had lost sight of the wonderful achievements of the last half-century. But she wasn't alone. In 2002, a UK government report began with the chilling comment that post-war optimism that we are about to conquer infectious disease "has proved dramatically unfounded". It continued, "At the beginning of the twenty-first century, infectious diseases are a major global threat: to health, to prosperity, to social stability, to security." The authors' anxiety was triggered by the fact that infectious diseases account for forty-one per cent of the disease burden around the world, with individual diseases such as HIV/AIDS, tuberculosis and malaria each killing millions of people every year.

As if to prove the point, in autumn 2005 emergency planners dusted off their 'flu pandemic contingency plans. A new version of influenza had hitch-hiked a lift on migratory birds and drifted from the Far East to Europe. Showing up in Russia had raised a few eyebrows. Arriving in Romania caused some concern, but the headline writers moved the story to the front pages, and politicians stammered for answers as the virus causing this disease killed birds in Greece. They found themselves staring down the barrel of a biological gun that could go off at any moment. Despite significant scientific know-how and complex medicine technology, we were cowering before one of the simplest biological entities on earth – a virus.

What went wrong? After all, it was way back in 1969 that the USA's Surgeon General William H. Steward optimistically testified before Congress that he was ready to "close the book" on infectious disease. His enthusiasm had been ignited by the plethora of antibiotics and vaccines that was appearing on the health market. Spurred on by similar hopes for Utopia, in 1977 the World Health Assembly set a goal. Their aim was that by the year 2000 governments and the World Health Organisation should enable all people of the world to have a level of health that would permit them to lead a socially and economically productive life. In 1981 this became the "Global Strategy for Health for All by the Year 2000" – the birth of the "Health for all" movement. While the WHO was keen to stress that this wouldn't mean the eradication of all disease, the implication was that we would soon enter an era of unprecedented good health; a new millennium, bringing a new age of hope.

If pride comes before a fall, complacency could precede calamity. Yes, beaming faces of super-health supermodels gaze at us from news stands and advertising billboards. Your colleagues arrive each morning with monotonous regularity, only rarely phoning in sick, and then on the whole they are back to their desks within a day or so – seldom more than a week. Health promotion literature tells us how to fine-tune our diets and lifestyles to squeeze an extra few years of activity into our lives. Campaigns are launched to try to stop our children overeating or damaging their otherwise good health with so-called recreational drugs.

Indeed, you would have to look hard in any Western society to find a person wandering around with untreated, festering sores. There may be one or two, but rushing by, living your own busy life, these people would easily be missed. Medical care in one form or another is available to all, even if you do have to wait a few hours in the emergency waiting room in order to receive it. Women enter the labour ward with the full expectation that they and their newborn child will leave a few hours or days later feeling sore and exhausted, but healthy. Life is good, and no-one is going to take it away from us.

So, living in the Western world it is easy to imagine that health for all is about to burst into reality. Science, it seems, has beaten disease into retreat – medicine is striding forward. Press stories each week confirm this view with more stories of breakthroughs and inventions. Infectious diseases that terrified our grandparents, such as measles, mumps and polio, are all but unheard of. And now that the book of life, the human genetic code, has been traced and recorded on computer discs, the remaining scourges of our time, diseases like cancer and heart disease, will soon join the list of afflictions beaten into submission. Things can only get better. Can't they?

It is an easy tactic to stir up a scare, but genuinely the answer may be

"No". Brundtland had real ground for anxiety. Our health-expecting sense of safety could be an illusion, or at best, under threat.

It's difficult for a generation that has received antibiotics and vaccinations from the first few weeks after emerging from the womb to come to terms with the fact that the war against disease is still on. Yes, there have been one or two clear victories, and a few cease-fires, and many microscopic foes may have been beaten into a retreat, but they are far from defeated. Disease-causing organisms, some so small that they can only be seen using the highest power microscopes currently available, are very much alive and kicking. No-one is safe.

"One out of every two people in low-income countries dies at an early age from an infectious disease. Most of these deaths should have been prevented," says Brundtland.[2] The WHO believes that an infectious disease crisis of global proportions is today threatening hard-won gains in health and life expectancy and infectious diseases kill some seventeen million people a year. That's more than 1,900 per hour. Before you get too complacent as you sit in your comfortable chair thinking that it's terribly sad, but living in the rich part of the world it won't affect me, take note that a third of these deaths occur in so-called developed countries. Heart disease and cancer may be the main killers in America, but infectious disease still accounted for twenty per cent of deaths in 1992.[3] This represents a fifty per cent increase since 1980. Respiratory infections, HIV and blood stream infections account for most of the increase.

In the USA approximately $120 billion, or fifteen per cent of the 1992 healthcare expenditure was directed at fighting infectious diseases, and hundreds of billions of dollars were forfeited through lost productivity.

Yes, a few battles have undoubtedly been won. If only every disease could be like the late smallpox. Smallpox was caused by a violent virus that first made itself apparent as the unwitting host developed an influenza-like illness accompanied by a rash that spread all over the victim's body. Forty per cent of infected adults and up to ninety per cent of children who caught the virus died a horrible death as the rash developed into pus-filled blisters and blindness and lung disease and kidney damage took hold. Those who survived were normally blind for life. Writing in the 1840s, English historian Thomas Macaulay paints a graphic picture of the disease: "The smallpox was always present, filling the churchyards with corpses, tormenting with constant fears all whom it had stricken, leaving on those whose lives it spared the hideous traces of its power, turning the babe into a changeling at which the mother shuddered, and making the eyes and cheeks of the big-hearted maiden objects of horror to the lover."[4]

In 1796 English physician Edward Jenner performed a vital experiment. Jenner was the third child of Reverend Stephen Jenner, vicar of Berkeley, Gloucestershire. At the age of thirteen he had become an apprentice to eminent surgeon Daniel Ludlow and aged twenty-one he joined John Hunter, the physician famous for pioneering surgery based on a careful study of anatomy. Two years later he returned to work in Gloucestershire and a further twenty-four years passed before he stepped into the history books. On May 14, 1796 he made two half-inch incisions on the surface of eight-year-old James Phipps' arm and spread cowpox matter over the wound. He had taken it originally from the hands of a milkmaid called Sarah Nelmes. Cowpox appeared to be similar to smallpox, but caused a less virulent disease, and folklore claimed that milkmaids who caught cowpox didn't get smallpox. Six weeks after giving the boy cowpox, Jenner exposed him to smallpox. I'm quite convinced that you would not get this bold experiment past a current research ethics committee, but the boy was fortunate. He did not become infected.

Jenner's controversial idea that exposure to a milder version of a disease could teach a person's body to fight full-scale onslaughts met severe opposition. The Royal Society rejected his manuscript describing the work on the basis that it was "in variance with established knowledge" and "incredible". Jenner was warned that he had "better not promulgate such a wild idea if he valued his reputation".[5] In the end he paid for his work to be published privately and a year later over seventy principal physicians and surgeons in London signed a declaration expressing their confidence in the idea. The concept of vaccination was born and the scene was set for smallpox to be driven into obscurity. Intriguingly, our language still remembers the event – the word vaccinate has its roots in the Latin *vacca*, meaning "cow".

By 1800 about 100,000 people had been vaccinated throughout the world. President Thomas Jefferson was one of the first key proponents of the method, appointing Benjamin Waterhouse, professor of the "Theory and Practice of Physic" at Harvard Medical School, as Vaccine Agent in the National Vaccine Institute.

In 1805 Napoleon had all his troops that had not had smallpox vaccinated and ordered the vaccination of all civilians a year later. In more recent history a world-wide effort co-ordinated by the World Health Organisation used mass vaccination programmes to weaken the disease's hold within whole populations, and drive it undercover. Then a medical rapid reaction force pounced on any minor outbreak that was reported. On March 2, 1971, two children were brought into the Eduardo Rabelo Hospital in Rio de Janerio. They had well-developed smallpox and their blisters were bursting, but they ended up being the last recorded cases of smallpox in the Americas. The final act in this macabre melodrama was played out in a small Somali village called Merka. On October 27, 1977, Ali Maow Maalin, a twenty-three-year-old hospital cook, took an infected child for treatment. Maalin caught the disease, but survived. The child died. The disease met its ignoble end. Or rather we thought it had and this should have been the end of the disease. Sadly, there was one last twist in the story that killed one more person – we'll meet her later.

Two years later, on Sunday December 9, 1979, the WHO's Global Commission for the Certification of Smallpox Eradication filed a report stating that smallpox was history. On May 8 the following year the report was presented to the World Health Assembly and accepted with acclamation.

New and Re-emerging Disease

Sadly, smallpox has proved to be the exception, rather than the rule. Old time diseases such as respiratory infections, diarrhoeal diseases, tuberculosis, malaria and measles still claim a total of 9.2 million people a year. These old battles are far from over.

Warfare is also breaking out on new fronts. Human Immunodeficiency Virus, better known as HIV, is continuing to ravage areas of Africa and is spreading rapidly in the East. It is a brand new agent, which brings with it the deadly disease of Acquired Immune Deficiency – AIDS. To all intents and purposes it is a new disease. It has similarities to a cat flu virus that has been around for many years, but no virus like this has ever attacked human populations. Its mode of transmission, which requires an exchange of blood or semen, means that when people are given correct health information they can avoid contracting it. But there is no reason why a new type of virus shouldn't emerge that could be spread in the airborne droplets shot at near supersonic speeds through our noses as we sneeze. After all, the common cold has succeeded in using this route of transmission for centuries.

Hepatitis C is another new kid on the block, having been identified only in 1989. Caused by a virus, infected people get flu-like symptoms first and then develop jaundice as their livers become inflamed. No tears form so their eyes dry and they feel extremely tired. Already estimates suggest that as many as 170 million people are infected with it. Like members of Britain's elite Special Air Services, who specialise in working undetected behind enemy lines, the virus uses a number of schemes to infiltrate the population. These include sexual contact, contaminated blood transfusions, poorly cleaned tattooing needles and hypodermic needles used repeatedly in some mass vaccinations or all too often shared by drug addicts.

If you don't know the subversive agent is there, your defensive systems are likely to be looking in the wrong direction. It begs the question, how many other diseases are moving stealthily through our population simply because we don't know of their existence?

Over the last couple of decades more than thirty diseases have been identified in humans for the first time. Some are believed to have emerged from rainforests and crossed the species barrier to infect humans. Others have seemingly had no previous history. HIV-AIDS is the classic example. Conspiracy theories and standard science make suggestions as to its origins, but no-one really knows.

Ebola haemorrhagic fever is another classic example of a horrendous disease with virtually no history. It first showed up at the beginning of the 1980s and then went back into hiding. In 1995 an outbreak in Zaire appeared to come from nowhere, but succeeded in killing three-quarters of the 316 people who became infected. About one third of the victims were healthcare workers who came into contact with blood or bodily fluids released from patients – the virus caused their insides to liquefy and then be coughed- and vomited-out as the victim perished.

Between November 1999 and March 2000, Marburg, a close relative of Ebola, attacked people in an area around a gold mine in the Democratic Republic of Congo. Sixteen died before the attack ended. More recently, between March and May 2005, at least 316 people in Angola were infected with Marburg. More than 270 of these victims died, giving the disease an impressive ninety per cent kill rate.

Dengue fever was relatively unheard-of forty years ago, but since then there has been a twenty-fold increase in the number of reported cases, with 514,139 cases being noted worldwide between 1990 and 1998. Lyme disease, hantavirus infection and foodborne *Escherichia coli* O157:H7 infection could also be added to the depressing list.

As if we didn't have enough to do looking out for newcomers, it seems that we are not doing very well keeping old enemies at bay. The Second World War will always be remembered as a scar on the twentieth century, but it was instrumental in causing many scientists to try to develop ways of fighting infections. The key breakthrough was the discovery that a chemical released from the mould *Penicillium notatum* could kill bacteria, but was not harmful to people. Antibiotics were harnessed, and with them came the hope of a magical world in which some of the worst diseases would melt away at the pop of a pill.

Tuberculosis was one of the first diseases to feel the heat, and over the middle years of the century it seemed to be disappearing from view. Unfortunately, the disease-causing organism has found a way of beating streptomycin, the antibiotic that performed the first wave of attack on TB and drove it almost into submission. Now once again the incidence of TB is soaring, especially among people whose own ability to fight infections has been weakened by other diseases like HIV-AIDS. Indeed, one of the first things that doctors look for if they suspect TB is to see whether HIV is also present.

On top of this, hospitals are in danger of becoming places where people get ill. A year 2000 report by the UK's Department of Health shows that almost one in ten people who go into a hospital for treatment become infected while they are there. As many as 5,000 people die as a direct result of that infection and a further 15,000 deaths could be partly attributable to the hospital bugs. Treating these infections costs an estimated £1 billion per year. The main culprit is *Streptococcus aureus*, an extremely common bacterium. About one third of the population have it lurking in crevices on their skin, but problems start if it gains entry to the body because then it can cause boils and blood poisoning.

The problem has been made worse as some of these critters have developed means of evading one of our most potent antibiotics, methicillin. These methicillin-resistant *Streptococcus aureus* (MRSA) bacteria are potentially lethal and are now believed to inhabit almost all of the hospitals in the UK, and a similar picture is found throughout the developed world. UK figures show that in 1998 there were 1,597 occasions when three or more people became infected by the same strain of bacteria in the same hospital in a single month.[6] In 2004, more than 3,500 people in hospitals around the UK became infected with MRSA, with MRSA bacteria found in the blood samples of more than 7,000 patients. Treating people without being able to resort to antibiotics is costly, time-consuming and, more importantly, is often unsuccessful.

In November 1999, Brian Duerden, the deputy director of Britain's Public Health Laboratory Service, warned that MRSA has reached "near epidemic" levels, saying that it is now held responsible for thirty-seven per cent of fatal cases of blood poisoning, compared to only three per cent eight years earlier. At the same time, Rosalind Plowman from the London School of Hygiene and Tropical Medicine claimed that reducing infections by just ten per cent could release £93.1 million, while saving 364,056 bed days.[7] The true figure could be about twice this number, as hospitals only record infections that manifest themselves while the patient is still in the ward. Those who acquire an infection in hospital, but only become ill once they get home, are not included in the statistics.

It is this upsurge in antibiotic resistance that caused a key chapter in a 1998 UK Department of Health report[8] to be entitled "Looking Into The Abyss". The report states that "in the closing years of the century, there is an uneasy sense that micro-organisms are 'getting ahead' and that therapeutic options are narrowing".[9] The basic problem is that there is a distinct possibility that we could run out of useful antibiotics. In similar tone, Joseph McCormick, a microbiologist working at the Institut Pasteur in Paris comments: "I cannot help but observe that we are swimming against a biological tide of overwhelming proportions, which is compounded by the lack of information from precisely those parts of the world where infectious diseases are highly endemic and populations rapidly expanding".[10]

Bacteria aren't the only killers that learn how to duck medical chemicals. The parasite at the heart of malaria has also shown itself remarkably capable of adapting. Initially quinine was a great solution, and was soon incorporated into a drink along with gin in an effort to disguise its bitter flavour, but within decades malaria was resistant to this drug. All further treatments aimed at preventing the bug gaining hold in a person have followed similar fates. So too have the attempts to rid the world of mosquitoes, the insect that transports malaria parasites from one animal or person to another. No sooner do you start to spray insecticides, than you find insects emerging that evolve biological defences and become resistant to the attack. The net consequence is that malaria is as damaging today as it has ever been, and growing populations in affected areas increases the human toll.

First Identify Your Enemy

Before you can begin a fight, you need to size up your opponent. Before you can do that you need to identify the subversive. Centuries of debate tried to grapple with the origin of disease, often seeing it in mystical or spiritual terms, without expecting to find a physical causal element. This debate took a new turn when in the 1800s the likes of French scientist Louis

Pasteur and German physician Robert Koch showed clearly that particles in the environment caused disease.

From the outset we need to be clear that there are a number of distinct classes of microscopic disease-causing bugs. Recognising the difference is important not merely from the point of view of classification, but because the different types need to be attacked in different ways.

Bacteria are one of the first groups to come to mind. They were first seen by the pioneering Dutch microscopist Anton van Leeuwenhoek, who built some 500 single-lens microscopes. Compared to modern microscopes, they were extremely simple devices. The lens was mounted in a tiny hole in the brass plate that made up the body of the instrument and the specimen was mounted on a sharp point that sticks up in front of the lens. Its position and focus could be adjusted by turning two screws. The entire instrument was only three to four inches long, and had to be held up close to the eye; it required good lighting and great patience to use.

All the same, in 1674 Leeuwenhoek began to observe bacteria and protozoa, referring to them as "very little animalcules". He found them almost everywhere he looked – rainwater, pond water and well water, and the human mouth and intestine. On September 17, 1683, the Royal Society published a formal paper that he had written describing the animalcules he had found on the plaque between his own teeth, "A little white matter, which is as thick as if "'twere batter". He repeated these observations on two other people, probably his wife and daughter, and on two old men who had never cleaned their teeth in their lives. Looking at these samples with his microscope, Leeuwenhoek reported how in samples from his own mouth he, "most always saw, with great wonder, that in the said matter there were many very little living animalcules, very prettily a-moving". The biggest sort "had a very strong and swift motion, and shot through the water (or spittle) like a pike does through the water". Other animalcules he noted "spun round like a top". In the material collected from old men he found "an unbelievably great company of living animalcules a-swimming more nimbly than any I had ever seen up to this time".

Bacteria had been recorded for the first time, but little did he know that some of them and their close relations would prove to be killers.

It took almost two hundred years before bacteria became associated with disease. In 1865, Louis Pasteur began to study the silkworm diseases that were crippling the silk industry in France. He discovered that micro-organisms were the infectious agents, a concept that became known as the "germ theory of disease". In so doing he dispelled the notion that organisms, including disease-causing organisms, spontaneously generate and proved that organisms reproduce new organisms. It proved to be one of the most important discoveries in medical history. With this knowledge, Pasteur was able to establish the basic rules of sterilisation, rules that revolutionised surgery and obstetrics.

As most people are well aware, the key feature about bacteria is that they can often be tackled by antibiotics. This is in marked contrast to viruses, which show no response to these bug-busting chemicals. It will be a recurrent theme through this book and I don't think it can be said too often.

Viruses are the second major class of infective agent. They are curious packages that can't really be described as being alive, because they have no power to operate on their own. In order to reproduce or to have any other effect, they need to gain entry into a cell and perform a *coup d'état* – taking control and setting up a fascist regime.

Spotting viruses is more difficult than bacteria because they are so small. They can get away with being so small because they don't carry around all the baggage needed to make a fully living organism. They are simply a parcel containing a code – and often that code has lethal consequences. The largest are about 450 nanometres (about 0.000014 inches) and the smallest are twenty nanometres (0.0000008 inches). Even using the most sophisticated light microscopes only the largest viruses can be seen.

It was in the 1840s that the German scientist Jacob Henle first postulated the existence of infectious agents too small to be seen with a light microscope, but for the lack of direct proof his hypothesis was not accepted. And although in the 1880s Louis Pasteur was working to develop a vaccine for rabies, a disease caused by a virus, he did not understand the concept of a virus.

During the last half of the nineteenth century, several key discoveries were made that set the stage for the discovery of viruses. The first experiment demonstrating viral infection was accomplished in about 1880. German scientist Adolf Mayer showed that extracts from infected tobacco leaves could transfer tobacco mosaic disease to a new plant, causing spots on the leaves. To his surprise, Mayer was unable to isolate a bacterium or fungus from the tobacco leaf extracts. He therefore concluded that tobacco mosaic disease might be caused by a soluble agent, but made the understandable mistake of thinking that the causal agent was a new type of bacterium.

The Russian scientist Dimitri Ivanofsky extended Mayer's observation. In 1892 he published work showing that the tobacco mosaic agent was small enough to pass through a porcelain filter that was so fine that it blocked all known bacteria. He too failed to isolate bacteria or fungi from the material that had passed through the filter. Like Mayer, Ivanofsky concluded that either the filter was defective or that the disease agent was a chemical that could dissolve into the solution – a toxin.

Unaware of Ivanofsky's results, the Dutch scientist Martinus Beijerinck, who collaborated with Mayer, performed his own filter experiment. He showed that the filtered material was not a toxin because it could grow and reproduce in the cells of the plant. In his 1898 publication, Beijerinck referred to this new disease agent as a contagious living liquid, *contagium vivum fluidum*, initiating a twenty-year controversy over whether viruses were liquids or particles.

The conclusion that viruses are particles came from several important observations. In independent studies in 1915 the British investigator Frederick Twort, and in 1917 the French-Canadian scientist Félix H. d'Hérelle, discovered a particular type of virus that infected bacteria. Félix H. d'Hérelle called them bacteriophage – eater of bacteria. In his experiment he grew a smooth sheet of bacteria on a culture plate and then washed it over with a solution containing the viral agent. Holes soon appeared in the culture. He concluded, correctly, that each hole occurred because a single viral particle had infected a bacterium, multiplied and destroyed all other bacteria in that region. This experiment provided the first method for counting infectious viruses (the plaque assay).

Then, in 1935, the American biochemist Wendell Meredith Stanley crystallised tobacco mosaic virus, demonstrating that viruses had regular shapes, and in 1939 tobacco mosaic virus was first visualised using the electron microscope.

For several decades viruses were referred to as filterable agents, and gradually the term virus (Latin for "slimy liquid" or "poison") was employed strictly for this new class of infectious agents.

Protozoa are the third class of merciless mercenaries. These microscopic multi-cellular animals often have extremely complex life histories, taking up residence in more than one type of host and adopting different physical forms as they move from one home to the next. Being relatively large, it would probably have been protozoa that Leeuwenhoek was often observing through his primitive microscope.

Malaria is one of the best known international criminals, and an example of a protozoal disease. The infective agent is one of four species of plasmodia – *Plasmodium falciparum*, *Plasmodium vivax*, *Plasmodium ovale* and *Plasmodium malariae*. Each of these spends part of its life living inside anopheline mosquitoes, and part living in the liver and red blood cells of mammals, often humans.

In fact malaria was the first disease to be attributed to a type of protozoa. In 1845, French pathologist Charles-Louis Laveran was born in Paris. He received his medical degree in 1867, and then became an Army surgeon. In 1879, Laveran started work in the military hospital of Bône in Algeria and in 1882 he moved to the malaria-infected marshy regions of Italy. His quest was to track down the causes of malaria, also known as marsh fever. Unlike other infectious diseases caused by bacteria, malaria's source was a medical mystery. Laveran studied blood samples and concluded that malaria was caused by parasites. His discovery gained formal recognition in 1889 and has since greatly contributed to the field of tropical medicine. In 1907, he was awarded a Nobel Prize for his work, and medical gun-sights started to be trained on protozoa.

You may go to the doctor expecting to be told you have a bacterial or viral infection, but I'm not sure how many people expect to find that they have been invaded by **fungi**. Most of the 100,000 species of fungi are either harmless or positively beneficial, but some four hundred of them are known to infect people, and the list is growing. They are responsible for problems ranging from mild irritation right the way through to death.

The agents that cause athlete's foot (*tinea*) or thrush (*candidiasis*) establish colonies on our skin, normally setting up shop where they find areas that are warm and moist. The inside of the mouth, the groin or vagina are particular favourites for thrush. It may not even be the fungus, but a fungal toxin that has an effect. *Aflatoxins*, for example, come from fungi that enjoy growing on peanuts. As the fungi grow they release a toxin and eating contaminated peanuts can result in a person's liver being damaged by that toxin.

The other way that these bugs cause damage is by releasing spores. These microscopic time capsules allow fungi to lay dormant for decades before finding themselves in the right environment and springing into life. Sadly for us, the protein that the spores are built of can often cause an allergic reaction if inhaled. For example, "farmer's lung" is caused by spores from mouldy hay. Where severe, the resulting lung-damage can lead to an early death.

Fungi don't only strike adults. In 1994, Dorr Dearborn from Case Western Reserve University in Cleveland, Ohio, was alerted to the danger of mould in homes when a thousand-fold increase in infant deaths from an unknown lung disease was reported. Between 1993 and 1998, Dearborn diagnosed thirty-seven cases of bleeding in the children's lungs.

Most were boys less than six months old. Thirty of the cases came from a small area of eastern Cleveland in Ohio. In November 1994, the USA's Centers for Disease Control and Prevention started a hurried investigation.

The finger of blame soon pointed at *Stachybotrys chartarum*, a fungus that thrives in damp wallpaper and wet cellulose-containing building materials. Tobacco smoke in the home seemed to be an accomplice in the crime. Now, Dearborn has set up a system whereby health inspectors visit homes before newborn babies leave the hospital. If there are signs of mould in the property, they find alternative accommodation for the family. In 1999, with this care plan in place, the incidence of disease has dropped to just one infected person.

But don't think the bug is beaten. Mould can turn up in every home, on windowsills and damp bathroom walls. In poorly built, or badly maintained homes, constant vigilance is needed to keep it at bay.

Infections that take hold in a person's body also have a remarkable way of becoming resistant to chemical agents spread in creams or sprays, or contained in tablets. Again these particular varieties of superbug take the easy route of knocking someone when they are down. Referred to as opportunistic infections, they occur in individuals whose defences are at a low ebb because of some disease like diabetes or HIV, or in people who are being treated for cancer or who have had an organ transplant.

Nellie Konnikov, Director of Dermatology Clinical Studies at Tufts University-New England Medical Center in Boston, told a conference in New Orleans of one such situation. A thirty-five-year-old white man with Hodgkin's disease had had a bone marrow transplant because he had lymphoma: a cancer that reduces the number of white blood cells designed to eat up dangerous bacteria. He received multiple courses of chemotherapy. On day eight, doctors noticed a few isolated red patches on his abdomen and they gave him amphotericin B, a drug that attacks fungal infections. Unfortunately, more red patches appeared all over his body and the skin in the spots started to die. Thirteen days after the first red patches appeared the patient died – his skin and lungs were riddled with a fungal infection.

The chances are that this poor man became infected by a bug that was lurking around the hospital. The USA's National Nosocomial Infections Surveillance Unit estimates that hospital-acquired infections affect more than two million patients each year, bearing a price tag of over $4.5 billion, and that the proportion of those infections caused by fungi rose from six per cent in 1980 to ten per cent in 1990.

Candida, the fungus that causes thrush, is the culprit in eighty per cent of those cases, but there are some nasty newcomers. Phaeohyphomycosis is a particularly nasty fungal disease. What starts as a minor prick, maybe on your finger, by a wood splinter, leads to a little raised, red patch that just won't heal. A fungus on the wood has established itself in the finger, and it's difficult to get out. The standard approach is to cut away the infected tissue and then treat the area with an anti-fungal drug. Why not just use the drug? Because no truly effective, knockout chemical against this bug exists in our armoury. It needs to be taken seriously because it is capable of causing large-scale damage. If you pick it up during a stay in hospital the effects can be severe, and some people have managed to get it into their brains, in which case the outlook is poor.

A Matter of Terms

It is worth taking a moment or two just to sort out a couple of terms – infectious and contagious.

A disease is infectious if it is caused by a specific micro-organism. Many diseases do not come into this category because, like eczema or skin cancer, they may be caused by exposure to a toxic chemical or radiation rather than a micro-organism. Other diseases are the result of faulty genetic codes in the centre of the person's cells.

An infectious disease is called contagious if it can be passed from one person to another by ordinary social contact, such as sharing a house or a workplace. The common cold, chickenpox and measles fit into this grouping. However, while HIV-AIDS and syphilis are infectious diseases, they are not called contagious because they need extra activities like sexual intercourse to pass them around.

Frontlines and Battlefields

Just as the enemy comes in many shapes and sizes, so the pathways and schemes used to evade our defences are varied. Micro-organisms thrive in almost every sector of the environment. Water and soil are loaded with them and many can survive for prolonged periods floating around in air if coughed or sneezed in an aerosol.

Water-borne disease is one of the most devastating, partly because so many people tend to rely on single sources of water. The world's worst outbreak of cryptosporidiosis, a severe diarrhoeal disease caused by a water-borne protozoa, occurred in April 1993 in Milwaukee, USA. Untreated water from a spring contaminated the local drinking water and out of the 800,000 people who relied on this particular source, some 370,000 became ill, 4,400 of whom had to go to hospital. Forty people are believed to have died as a result of the infection.

The other problem is one of numbers and dilution. One person with cholera excretes 10^{13} bacteria each day – that's ten million million. Now you only need to ingest about a million of these bacteria in order to become infected, so one person could infect up to ten million others every day. In the case of *Campylobacter* the effect could be more drastic because the infective dose is five hundred cells and *Shigella* requires only two hundred cells to make you very ill.

If these numbers make you feel uneasy in the water, then don't think you are safe on the land. There are plenty of bugs in the soil just waiting to get you. Some parts of the world, particularly areas around Afghanistan, are riddled with anthrax, a disease that primarily affects plant-eating animals. It's not fussy though and will quite happily take on human beings as well. The bacteria involved, *Bacillus anthracis*, gets in via a small cut in your skin, or hitches a lift on flying particles of dust as it is sucked into your lungs. One in five people who are infected can expect to die as black blisters break out on their skin and the blood becomes loaded with toxic chemicals. Anthrax bacteria also have a nasty habit of forming spores, and these can lay dormant in the earth for years and decades... just waiting for you.

It was with a huge sense of relief that doctors found that HIV couldn't travel through the air. The virus is devastating enough, even though it can move only via body fluids such as blood and semen. On the other hand the viruses behind the common cold find nothing easier. Sneeze into the air, and they are off to find their next host. Shake hands with someone who has just sneezed into a tissue or worse still into their hand and not washed it, and then rub or pick your nose, or suck your finger, and you will have been got. It's that simple.

The other trick employed is to get a bigger animal to carry you to your victim. We have already seen that malaria protozoa make use of mosquitoes, but this is far from an isolated case. Plague, a disease notorious for wiping out fifty million people, one third of Europe's population in the mid-1300s, makes use of a flea that lives on a rat. Lyme disease is caused by the bacterium *Borrelia burgdorferi*, and this bug is transmitted by the bites of ticks that usually live on deer, but can also make themselves perfectly at home on dogs.

Machupo virus, a bug so rare that has only ever been seen in one epidemic site in Bolivia, makes use of mouse urine to get about. Once it gets into humans the effect is phenomenal. Survivors describe how they drift in and out of consciousness. Every touch is agony, to the extent that they can't even bear the pressure of a sheet. Their eyes become a shocking red as blood leaks into them and small rivulets of fluid leak out of microscopic holes all over the victim's skin. Unsurprisingly, half of the people who pick up this particular bug die.

Of Planes and People

Two aspects of contemporary human existence have served to move the issue of unstoppable disease up the international political and scientific agenda – international travel and mega-cities.

Flying into an airport in Australia is a strange experience. Bleary-eyed after a long flight you are then challenged by the cabin stewards striding down the corridors spraying a can of insecticide from each hand. Why? To kill off unwanted passengers in the form of stowaway insects that might escape and establish unwanted colonies. I've never been convinced that it is desperately effective, partly because some of the worst diseases travel in the guts and blood streams of passengers, but it proves a point. Aircraft are perfect ways of transporting microbiological criminal elements to new destinations.

Also the sheer numbers of international journeys is increasing. Between 1993 and 1997 the volume of international arrivals into the Americas increased by thirty-two per cent, those arriving in Europe went up by twenty-seven per cent and the figures for Africa and the Middle East show a forty-five per cent increase. There were two million passengers in 1950 and 1.4 billion at the turn of the millennium.

It is not just arriving that is the problem. The travelling can be just as dangerous, as people are packed into small spaces sharing re-circulated air. I regularly come down with a cold after a trans-Atlantic flight, but that's nothing when compared to the seventy per cent of passengers on a single flight held on the ground in the United States for a couple of hours in 1977 who came down with an identical 'flu bug.

Even if the flight takes off, you can still be in trouble. In March 2003, the virus that causes the respiratory disease SARS became a microscopic stowaway on a three-hour flight from Hong Kong to Beijing. The virus had infected one passenger, but as it was breathed into the cabin air it managed to take up new lodgings in up to eighteen other passengers. Some of the newly infected people were sitting as many as seven rows away from the carrier. This incident raises questions about how frequently cabin air should be circulated through the plane's air conditioning system, and how often it should be changed. Assuming everything is working properly, air should be cycled every two or three minutes, with half of the old air being thrown away and replaced with fresh on each cycle. This in itself removes half of the bugs, and filters in the air system of those planes which have them will clear even more.

The issue comes down to balancing economics and risk. It takes energy to filter the air and to grab new oxygen from outside the cabin. Energy costs money. The question becomes how much more are we prepared to pay for our plane tickets in order for the airline to reduce the risk of our catching an airborne disease? A 2005 review of air travel concluded that in an ideal world air should be circulated twice as fast as it is now, but experts believe that if this change added £20 to a ticket people would be likely to vote with their feet and fly with a less safe competitor.

That said, don't get complacent and spend your day in a departure lounge. The air there is far staler, and still full of the same bugs you will encounter on board.

Planes aren't alone in carrying bugs. In 1985, the aggressive tiger mosquito slipped unnoticed into the United States inside a shipment of water-logged tyres that had just arrived from Asia. Within two years the mosquitoes had established themselves in seventeen states, bringing with them their payload of yellow fever, dengue and other diseases.

Early in 1991, so the theory goes, a Chinese ship docked near Chancay, a coastal district of Peru just north of the capital, Lima. Unknown to its crew, the water in its sewage tanks was contaminated with the bacteria that causes cholera. The people of Peru soon found out, because when it was discharged into the sea the bacteria sparked off an epidemic that spread rapidly through South and Central America. Hundreds of thousands of people became infected and some eleven thousand people died.

One reason why the epidemic was so devastating directs our attention to the other current crisis – mega-cities with large, poor populations. Cholera is unpleasant to get, but it shouldn't kill. Dehydration caused by diarrhoea is the key issue, but if the person can get access to plenty of clean water they will get well. People living in poverty often don't have that luxury. In addition, these people are packed together like so many sardines in a tin. This is a perfect scenario for bugs to jump from person to person, maybe with the assistance of poor sewage and poor personal hygiene.

The Armoury

So what are the weapons at our disposal? The hundreds of chemical agents now available can be good at tackling bacteria, protozoa and fungi, but there are only a few examples of agents that have any success attacking viruses. Certainly, antibiotics are useless. This is because while antibiotics take out some of the biochemical processes inside the bacteria, viruses are primitive particles and therefore don't have any processes to tamper with.

Vaccines are the other main tool. These boost the person's immune system, fooling it into thinking that it has just been infected by the disease-causing agent. If at any point in the future the real bug does gain entry into the body, then the immune system will be ready and waiting and will be able to mount a rapid response, hopefully destroying the agent before it causes any problems.

One thing will become clear as we go through this book, however, and that is that bugs are good at learning. No sooner do you have one antibiotic, than they learn to by-pass it. Just as you develop a vaccine, they tend literally to change their coat so that the vaccine has reduced effectiveness.

At the end of the day, the best defence we have is good old hygiene. Wash your hands, breathe fresh air, drink clean water and eat fresh, appropriately cooked food. It is much better to avoid, rather than fight, an infection.

Superbugs Are Go

There is nothing new about infectious bugs. There is equally nothing new about bugs that appear to have the upper hand. What is new is that in the last few decades we have become remarkably relaxed about them and treat them casually.

Bugs are here. Their big brothers, the superbugs, come in a host of shapes and sizes. Some have been the target of our systems of medicine and hygiene for centuries, others we are just discovering. Some old enemies are learning new tricks. We need to learn from history, look after the present and plan for a future that gives them the respect they deserve.

CHAPTER 2 –
LESSONS FROM HISTORY

Travelling is a rewarding activity. But stay in one place, share your life with just one particular set of people, and you could soon get the impression that your lifestyle and sense of priorities are shared by everybody else. Television has done a bit to shatter this illusion. People in wealthy countries get a glimpse of life without technology and all too often adopt a patronising attitude, saying that technology would ruin their simple existence. Those who have few possessions are increasingly making a television and satellite dish an early purchase if cash comes their way. They see programming that sells an equally distorted illusion of life in the wealthy West.

If you really want to know, there is no option but to get out, see people in different cultures and experience other ways of organising a society. And once the dust has settled and the aspects of life that unnerved you when you arrived have subsided, you quickly find that there are some underlying principles that haven't changed. There is the desire to be loved and the need to care for others. There is the need to earn a living and the requirement to keep as well as is possible.

The same, I am sure, would be true if you could travel in time, rather than space. If you could step back a few centuries you would find people living out their existence with similar goals, but their priorities and expectations would be different. Much of this difference would stem from the fact that good health would be seen as a bonus, not an expectation. For someone living in the cosy well-off regions of the world, the experience would be valuable because it would give a flavour of the uncertainty that currently faces the majority population of our world – people for whom good health is not taken for granted. It would also paint a picture of the sort of world that we could return to if we ever let infectious diseases get the upper hand. As we will see, it is not wanton scaremongering to suggest that that could happen.

Plague

Plague makes a good place to start. Not just because it has a vivid history, but because it has an all too colourful present.

Plague seems to be one of the oldest recorded diseases, indeed it could be the devastating illness recorded in the Old Testament of the Bible (1 Samuel 6) that struck the Philistines after they had stolen the Ark of the Covenant. The manuscripts talk of tumours that killed the people being associated with a great number of rats.

The causal agent in plague is a bacterium, *Yersinia pestis*. The bug was first isolated by French bacteriologist Andre Yersin in 1894. We now know that there are three different biotypes of this rod-shaped bacterium (*Antiqua*, *Orientalis* and *Mediaevalis*), but they differ only in the fine detail of the way they obtain energy from food, not in the manner of the disease they cause. The bacteria tend to live in rodent populations and are transmitted from one to another by fleas. Fortunately for the bacteria, but unfortunately for us, rodents appear to be relatively resistant to the disease. The fleas only move over to human hosts if the rats they were living on die in such numbers that they run out of homes, or if the people have to live in very close proximity to the rats. The classic flea that is normally blamed for this is the oriental rat flea, *Xenopsylla cheopis*, but the bug isn't fussy and can be transmitted by any one of over 1,500 flea species.

When a flea draws blood from an infected rat, *Y. pestis* is drawn into its gut. At each feed the flea takes between 0.03 and 0.5 microlitres of blood, a tiny drop; but it's loaded with bugs. At temperatures below 27°C the bacteria grow, but become clumped together, blocking the flea's gut. The flea becomes hungry and feeds often. Each time it bites a new host, however, the flea's stomach contents, including the bacteria, are vomited into the host's blood. Another animal or person just became infected. Intriguingly, at environmental temperatures greater than 27°C the bacteria still grow, but the gut remains clear. With a flow of food through its gut, the flea is less hungry. Add the two factors together and the number of bacteria released is diminished because they feed less often and don't regurgitate with each bite. As a consequence, transmission is less likely to happen in summer months than in the winter. However, *unlikely* does not mean that it *won't*.

Once infected, symptoms appear within one to seven days. There are three forms of the plague, all caused by the same bacterium. The bubonic form is characterised by large buboes, swollen lymph nodes in the neck, armpits or groin. Sometimes an ulcer or purulent spot develops at the site where the flea bit. Bubonic plague victims characteristically flex and extend their arms in attempts to lessen the pain of the buboes. Infection of the blood can lead to bleeding beneath the skin, which causes the characteristic black splodges on the skin. These symptoms are accompanied by a very high fever, headache, shaking chills and delirium and are followed by death in fifty to sixty per cent of cases when left untreated.

Bubonic plague bacterium can infect a person's lungs, causing the pneumonic form of the disease. Pneumonic plague is highly contagious, being spread person-to-person via aerosolised, bug-packed droplets. No need for fleas this time. Victims of pneumonic plague develop a severe cough and expel bloody sputum. Pneumonic plague leads to a coma and death in almost all cases if treatment isn't started within hours of the first symptoms.

The third form of plague is the septicaemic form. This occurs when massive quantities of *Y. pestis* get into the victim's bloodstream, causing rashes, gangrene and death within a day. Blood clotting, multiple organ failure and difficulty breathing make this version of the disease almost one hundred per cent fatal.

The Roman Empire was famous for setting up systems of rapid transport. Straight roads blasted their way across continents and a new-found safety allowed merchants to roam far and wide. It also allowed flea-ridden rodents to move to new territories. In 540 AD, during the reign of Emperor Justinian, a pandemic (an epidemic that spreads across whole continents) broke out in Pelusium, Lower Egypt, and spread through Alexandria and on to Palestine. From there it travelled the world. At the peak of the crisis, estimates suggest that ten thousand people were dying each day. Maybe one hundred million people died in all. Historians say that this scourge contributed to the fall of the Roman Empire.

The winter of 1347 was a bad time to live in Europe. It was a particularly bad time to live in England, where the pandemic became dubbed the "Black Death", either because of the black spots it produced on the skin, or the blackening colour of limbs as the tissue started to die. The historic origin of the pandemic seems to have been China, but since China was a principal trading nation, it was only a matter of time before the outbreak would occur. In October 1347, several merchant ships arrived from the Black Sea port of Caffa, one of the key links in trade with China. When the ships docked in Messina, Sicily, many of those on board were already dead and the rest were dying of plague. Within days the disease spread to the city and the surrounding countryside.

Eyewitness accounts describe how fathers abandoned sons and lawyers refused to come out and make wills for the dying. Friars and nuns were left to care for the sick, but it wasn't long before the monasteries and convents were deserted, as they too were stricken. Bodies lay in their houses as there was no-one left to bury them. The Italian writer Giovanni Boccaccio described how victims "ate lunch with their friends and dinner with their ancestors in paradise".

The plague was not limited to a certain group of people. Everyone could catch it. The rich had an advantage over the poor in that they could escape the putrid cities and run away to their country castles and villas. The country was less crowded and had a smaller rat population so they were safer – but by no means free from danger. The poor had no money to flee with and no work to do if they did leave the cities, so they stayed and perished.

Between seventeen and fifty-five million people were wiped out. This was from a total European population of one hundred and fifty million. Some communities lost ninety per cent of their population. Society disintegrated as people fled from towns to seek places of isolation. They realised that transport was a potential threat and some ports instigated a system whereby ships were isolated for forty days before anyone was allowed to disembark – they were placed in "quarantine".

Even when the worst was over, smaller outbreaks continued through to the 1600s. So many people died that medieval society never recovered. Serious labour shortages throughout Europe led to workers' demands for higher wages. Landlords refused the demands and revolts broke out across the Continent.

The Great Plague of London in 1665 was one of the last major historic outbreaks. At its peak it killed seven thousand people per week, wiping out a third of London's half a million population. The disease disappeared in 1666 when a vast area of London was destroyed in a single fire – the Great Fire of London.

The third pandemic began in Canton and Hong Kong in 1894 and spread rapidly throughout the world, carried by rats aboard the swifter steamships that replaced slow-moving sail vessels. By 1903, plague had entered seventy-seven ports on five continents – thirty-one in Asia, twelve in Europe, eight in Africa, four in North America, fifteen in South America and seven in Australia. Some thirteen million people died in India alone.

Since then the western third of the United States has had incidences of plague, including Oregon in 1934, Utah in 1936, Nevada in 1937, Idaho 1940, New Mexico in 1949, Arizona in 1950, Colorado in

1957 and Wyoming in 1978. The low population density in North America as a whole seems, however, to have saved it from a widespread epidemic. So, while plague is very much a part of the world's history, it is also part of the present. Two hundred and forty-seven cases of human plague have been reported and thirty-seven patients have died in the US between 1980 and 1997, the highest of any eighteen-year period since the early 1900s.

In South America in recent years human plague has been reported in Bolivia, Brazil, Ecuador and Peru. In Africa there have been reports of plague from Angola, Botswana, Democratic Republic of the Congo (Zaire), Kenya, Libya, Madagascar, Malawi, Mozambique, South Africa, Tanzania, Uganda, Zambia and Zimbabwe. In Asia, China, India, Kazakhstan, Laos, Mongolia, Myanmar (Burma) and Vietnam have reported cases.

Far from dying out, the disease seems to be holding its own, with three periods of increased activity in the last half of the twentieth century – the mid-1960s, 1973–1978 and the mid-1980s. The latest figures for 1997 show one of the highest recorded levels in recent history with 4,370 reported cases and 154 deaths. The WHO believes this is probably a gross underestimate of the real situation. In the United States reported cases have increased from three in the 1950s to thirteen in the 1990s.

However, the chief cause for concern is that we might be on the verge of becoming incapable of curing the disease once a person becomes infected. Antibiotics, the mainstay in tackling bacterial infections, are losing their effectiveness, and a 1997 report in the *New England Journal of Medicine*[1] sent shivers down the spine. In 1995, a sixteen-year-old boy living in the Ambalavao district of Madagascar had come into hospital with fever, chills and painful muscles. Doctors initially thought he had malaria, but three days after he arrived, a bubo appeared on the inside of his thigh. His temperature soared and he became delirious.

Alerted by the bubo, his doctors started treating him for plague. Plague arrived in the island nation of Madagascar in 1898, probably aboard steamships from India. Vaccination campaigns, improved hygiene and the discovery of antibiotics and insecticides brought the disease under control. Between 1950 and 1980 there were only twenty to fifty cases per year among the five million people who live in the infected plains in the centre of the island and the west coast port of Mahajanga. Since 1989 the numbers have started to rise with over two thousand suspected cases in some years.

The acquired wisdom is that treatment is relatively straightforward. Just give antibiotics. Chloramphenicol, streptomycin and tetracyclin are the recommended combatants. Because the disease was advanced, his doctors gave him a cocktail using streptomycin and a less commonly used trimethoprim-sulfamethoxazole. The boy recovered.

As part of a standard surveillance program the hospital staff, along with members of the WHO's Collaborating Centre for Yersinia at the Institut Pasteur, Paris, and the Plague Central Laboratory in Antananarivo, the capital of Madagascar, tested samples of the infective agent. It was then that their hearts must have missed a beat. The particular bacterium that had infected this boy proved to be resistant to almost all antibiotics; it just happened to be knocked on the head by the trimethoprim-sulfamethoxazole they had used – fortunately for the patient.

How the bacteria had managed to get hold of the genetic information that they needed to be capable of resisting this vast spectrum of antibiotics remains something of a mystery. But the fact that they could set international alarm bells ringing. This particular bug showed up in a part of the world where doctors are used to looking for the symptoms. It was also fortunate that there was a hole in its resistance armoury. But neither of those two features is guaranteed. The next resistant bug to come along may have a fully comprehensive coverage, and tourism or trade could introduce it into naïve areas. The possibility should not be neglected or ignored. You can only begin to imagine the effect of a resistant version of pneumonic plague in a densely populated country. Certainly, I wouldn't want to be an eyewitness.

In reporting the incident, the medics concluded that "the observation that Y. pestis is able to acquire, under natural conditions [multidrug resistance], regardless of its true origin, indicates that such a clinically ominous event may occur again". David Dennis of the Centers for Disease Control and Prevention's division of vector-borne infectious disease in Fort Collins, Colorado, commented, "It's sort of a wake-up call to the international community that deals with emerging disease, and plague in particular, that we need to be on alert for the possibility of emergence of drug resistance in plague strains". Commenting on this in an editorial in the New England Journal of Medicine, Dennis and colleague James Hughes point out that this provides "another grim reminder that emerging infectious diseases and anti-microbial resistance in one location can pose serious problems for the entire world... The finding of multidrug-resistant Y. pestis in Madagascar reinforces the concern expressed by an Institute of Medicine committee that the threat from the emerging infectious diseases is not to be taken lightly."[2]

Smallpox

More than two hundred years ago, Edward Jenner performed an experiment that laid the foundation for the apparent eradication of smallpox. This viral disease has a long history, however, and one that has lessons to teach us.

The Spread of Dread

Historians believe that the disease appeared when people in north-eastern Africa started to develop settled agriculture, as opposed to nomadic hunter-gatherer lifestyles, in around 10,000 BC. Faces of mummies from the eighteenth and twentieth Egyptian Dynasties (1570–1085 BC) have classical smallpox marks, as does the well-preserved mummy of Ramses V, who died as a young man in 1157 BC.

The first recorded smallpox epidemic occurred in 1350 BC, during the Egyptian-Hittite war. The virus probably passed to the Hittite population from Egyptians they had taken captive. All were at risk – soldiers and civilians, rich and poor. The Hittite King Suppiluliumas I and his heir, Arnuwandas, both fell victim to the disease, and their civilisation fell into sharp decline. Egyptian merchants took it along with their trade to India in the last millennium BC.

Jenner may be recorded in European history as the pioneer who saved the world from this ghastly disease, but the roots of his success were planted during the epidemic in Athens in 430 BC when Greek historian Thucydides noted that those who survived the disease were later immune to it. These observations were reiterated by the ninth century Persian physician Rhazes, who in 910 AD wrote the first detailed description of smallpox, *De Variolis Et Morbillis Commentarius*. Rhazes also noted that the illness was transmitted between people and distinguished the disease from measles.

Between 165 and 180 AD an outbreak of smallpox raged in the Roman world, killing between 3.5 and 7 million people in Marcus Aurelius' empire. The disease appears to have been brought to Rome by an army which picked it up while fighting the Parthians in an area now part of Iran. The army was severely weakened by the infection and beat a hasty retreat, with the survivors spreading the disease around the Mediterranean basin as they fled. The Arab expansion, the Crusades and the discovery of the West Indies all contributed to its globalisation. The disease arrived in the New World when Spanish and Portuguese explorers set foot on the continent. The effect on this previously unexposed population was extreme and it was one of the diseases that contributed to the fall of the Aztec and Inca empires.

A similar story is told for the eastern coast of North America, where the advent of smallpox decimated the native population. The slave trade made matters worse by introducing the disease straight from its point of origin in Africa.

Smallpox was no respecter of wealth or power, and most countries seem to have lost a key figure at some point over the past five hundred years. In 1646 it killed Prince Baltasar Carlos, heir to the Spanish throne, and in 1650 William II of Orange and his wife, Henrietta, fell to its power. Emperor Ferdinand IV of Austria died of it in 1654, and just to prove that it wasn't only vindictive against Europeans, Emperor Gokomyo of Japan died of the disease in the same year. China lost her Emperor, Fu-lin, in 1661 and England lost her Queen Mary II in 1694. King Nagassi of Ethiopia died in 1700, and Tsar Peter II of Russia in 1730. Scandinavia wasn't spared as Ulrika Eleanora, Queen of Sweden, died of the pox in 1741.

The power to kill seems to have varied between twenty and sixty per cent. Survivors normally bore disfiguring scars and corneal infection left many survivors blind. Infants were at particular risk. In the 1700s some eighty per cent of infected children below the age of five living in London succumbed, and ninety-eight per cent of those in Berlin.

Variolation to the Rescue

The only thing that could make you safe from smallpox was to catch it and survive to tell the story. Realising this, some people in the 1600s started to take the risky step of deliberately infecting themselves, hoping that they could control the extent of the infection, get only a mild version of the disease, and become immune. Various methods of so-called "variolation" (variola being another name for smallpox) were used, including spreading scabs or pus from scabs on the person's skin. Some people scraped the skin beforehand to enhance uptake. Another technique was to blow the powdered scabs of smallpox pustules into the nostrils.

Variolation came to Europe at the beginning of the eighteenth century although the English physicians were very sceptical. It took the enthusiasm of Lady Mary Wortley Montagu to start to get the technique accepted in England. Her desire to find a solution was driven by her personal experience of the horrors of the disease, which had disfigured her reputably beautiful face in 1715. The disease had also killed her twenty-year-old brother eighteen months earlier. While on official duties, she witnessed old women performing the technique in Istanbul and worked hard to ensure that as many people knew of the technique as possible.

The problem with variolation lay in the fact that real smallpox viruses were being used. Consequently two to three percent of variolated people died of smallpox. On occasion these victims even became the source of a new epidemic. All the same, it was deemed a better risk than not doing it – but the risk was tangible.

To a Safer World

The route to a safe vaccine came from the realisation that exposure to a different, but loosely related disease, could trigger protection. The disease in question was cowpox.

Some one hundred years before Edward Jenner's work, Chinese physicians developed a system in which they compacted fleas taken from cows, making them into tablets. Swallowing these pills was therefore the first recorded example of oral vaccination. The system worked because the fleas had ingested tiny amounts of cowpox-containing blood, so the tablets contained small doses of the cowpox virus, a close relative of smallpox, and it was cowpox that Jenner, who himself was variolated at the age of eight, made use of.

Jenner didn't dream up the idea, he "simply" investigated it thoroughly and published the results. In scientific research, publication becomes associated with the origination and ownership of the idea. In 1802 Jenner wrote that he believed that this idea could annihilate smallpox.[3] It took almost two hundred years, but as we have heard, it happened.

Or has it? Why does the WHO recommend that half a million vials of smallpox vaccine are kept in storage, if smallpox has been eradicated? Why has the US just started to manufacture new stocks of the vaccine? Two answers. First, absence of evidence is not evidence of absence. Just because no one has got ill with the disease is not proof that every last virus has disappeared. There might be one locked up in some part of the world, just waiting to find its way into an unsuspecting person. The WHO believes that this is unlikely – very unlikely – but not quite impossible.

Secondly, not all the known viruses have been destroyed. The samples held in labs in the US and Russia are the real thing. If poor management or inappropriate handling occurred, they could break out of their secure lab. Then we would be in trouble. After all, virtually no-one in the world is currently vaccinated against this bug so it would have a field day. The vaccines are a safety net.

Before you think that I am introducing a cheap scare, consider this. In 1978, the year after the last natural case of smallpox, Janet Parker died of the disease. She was a medical photographer working in the University of Birmingham's Medical School. Her office was one floor above the laboratory where smallpox was being stored. Professor Henry S. Bedson, head of the Department of Medical Microbiology, subsequently committed suicide after an investigation revealed that the air duct system was improper, and that researchers frequently left gowns on after leaving the smallpox laboratory. Approximately three hundred people had to be quarantined, but in the end only Parker's mother developed smallpox and she survived. It is just this sort of incident that could let the bug loose.

The Final Curtain...

So if the only known viruses are in captivity, why not destroy them and be done with it? One argument claims that it is environmental vandalism knowingly to drive any biological entity into oblivion, even a nasty one. If we start with smallpox, the argument goes, where will we stop given that plenty of other species are unpleasant?

However, a more powerful case has been made for not destroying it yet on the basis that we might be able to learn a lot of useful tips from studying it. Viruses could be tamed and harnessed as valuable medical tools. Given that smallpox is so successful, it might show us some unique tricks. By destroying the last few examples of it we could lose that information.

Four deadlines have been set for its destruction. Three have passed – December 31, 1993, June 30, 1995 and June 31, 1999 – with smallpox being granted a last-minute stay of execution on each occasion. The deadline set for 2002 became the deadline for the scientists to set a deadline and this lapsed with no serious action. For the first pioneers of smallpox eradication this delay must seem incomprehensible. What could we possibly learn from these lethal particles of biology that is so valuable it is worth taking the risk, however small, of allowing the disease to escape Houdini-like from the lab and run amok?

The answer lies in the information that scientists are generating by studying this agent of destruction. When geneticists decoded the genetic material inside the smallpox virus they had a shock. To start with the code sequence is huge. The virus contains one hundred and eighty-six thousand base pairs of DNA (letters of code), which contains the information for about one hundred and eighty-seven genes. This makes smallpox one of the most complicated viruses known. But what startled the researchers was that many of the viral genes showed great similarities to bits of human genetic code. Some one hundred of these genes give instructions for key parts of the human immune system, giving a clue as to why smallpox is so lethal. Packaged inside its tiny coat, the virus has an insider's knowledge of the defensive strategies of its desired host – us. It's like giving a bank-robber the combination numbers that disarm the security systems.

Studying smallpox, the scientists insist, could give us valuable clues about how to fight diseases where a person's immune system goes wrong – diseases like diabetes and rheumatoid arthritis. It could lead to an under-standing of how other viruses, including HIV and Ebola, commit their deadly crimes. Who knows? The final chapter in the history of smallpox might even tell us that it has been tamed and is now roaming the wards saving lives.

So, for the moment, smallpox looks safe. Photographs of current victims no longer fill pages of newspapers, nor do they occupy hours of broadcast time, so no-one is particularly worried about it. But remember: the disease might be dead, but the virus "lives" on. And in a world concerned with the threat of bioterrorism there is now the fear that it could fall into the wrong hands.

Syphilis

The politics of naming a disease is intriguing. Venetian, Naples and French disease were all names given at one time or another to what is now called syphilis, as people have tried to blame each other for the arrival of the scourge. One possibility that is currently gaining acceptance is that, in a reverse of smallpox, this is one disease that the Americas gave to Europe.

Syphilis is caused by a spiral-shaped bacterium called *Treponema palladium*, which gains entry through broken skin or the mucus membranes in the genitalia. These bugs are readily transmitted by direct skin-to-skin contact. Sharing a drinking vessel is enough, kissing will do, but on the whole it is sexual intercourse that is the main means of acquiring an infection.

The disease causes a one-centimetre painless ulcer that usually develops on the person's genitals. This site tends to heal within six to eight weeks. A month or so later a rash breaks out and things become decidedly more unpleasant. Headaches, aching bones, loss of appetite, fever and fatigue can all set in, and the person's hair comes out in clumps. If not treated, this can last for years. A few people go on to develop bone damage and soft tissue damage that can even lead to dementia.

For years academics have debated whether the natives of the Americas gave the disease to the settlers, or if it was another way around. Others suggest that it originated on both sides of the Atlantic. After all, the first clear descriptions of syphilis only occur in the early 1500s, a few years after Columbus' famed October 12, 1492 landing. The search for the truth lies in the bones. Checking skeletons from people who lived and died before this date shows which populations were affected.

The most likely answer is that a version of syphilis existed in the New World prior to 1492, and other similar bugs were present in Europe. The outbreak that spread across Europe at the beginning of the sixteenth century quite possibly resulted from the New World and Old World versions coming together and sharing their genetic endowment.

Syphilis appears to teach us that travelling not only brings the possibility of introducing a new disease to a new area. It also creates the opportunity for previously separated, mildly potent bugs to meet up and engender a new, nastier version.

Polio

Spurred on by their excitement over ridding the world of smallpox, the WHO has turned its attention to polio. It's a good candidate. Like smallpox, polio is caused by a virus that can live only in humans. This means that you don't have to go around driving it out of huge populations of wild animals, you can concentrate on *Homo sapiens*. There is also a vaccine that can give people immunity. In addition, the disease is sufficiently gruesome to warrant the billions of dollars that have already been spent, and will need to be spent, if the task is going to be completed.

Polio, an abbreviated name for poliomyelitis, usually causes only a mild illness. The virus normally lives in the gut and is excreted in faeces. On occasion, however, it penetrates the gut lining and attacks the brain and spinal cord, wrecking nerves and thus paralysing some muscles. If the muscles involved in breathing are affected the person has a high chance of dying. In the past these people were often nursed in iron lungs – huge bath tub-like cases that allowed the patient's head to stick out through a rubber seal at one end. A pump then forced air into and out of the iron lung, increasing and decreasing the pressure surrounding the patient's chest and helping them to breathe.

Polio has probably killed people throughout the whole of human history. A three thousand-year-old Egyptian stone engraving shows an identifiable reference to paralytic polio. However, recorded cases are rare in ancient times, but they started to increase as sanitation became better. Once houses had indoor plumbing, and sewage systems kept waste away from drinking water, babies were no longer exposed to the virus and so didn't develop immunity to it. Going to school or swimming in the local baths then exposed them to danger.

An epidemic in the north-eastern United States in the summer of 1916 killed six thousand people – mostly children – and left twenty-seven thousand people with some form of disability. There were serious epidemics in 1936, 1937, 1941, 1944, 1946, 1949, 1951, 1952 and 1954.

With the advent of a vaccine the disease has been forced into a retreat. In the UK in 1955 there were 6,331 cases, but this has dropped rapidly to just four cases in 1985. There have been no cases in recent years. In the USA the story is similar, as it killed two thousand people in 1955 and paralysed a further sixteen thousand, but had been banished by 1994.

With numbers of cases dropping around the world, the WHO launched an eradication program in 1988. At that point there were still thirty-five thousand cases worldwide per year, with most of these occurring in Africa and Asia. By 1998, with eighty-two per cent of the world's children vaccinated, the WHO initiative had reduced the numbers of cases to 3,200 and the target is to complete the task by 2005. The grim reaper would appear to be poised to collect polio.

But just as the WHO is thinking about sending out joyful press releases, there are a few murmurs that urge caution. One of the loudest comes from Paul Fine who works at the London School of Hygiene and Tropical Medicine. His anxiety stems from the fact that the vaccine employed in this campaign makes use of a weakened live polio virus. It's the vaccine that is either dripped into the person's mouth, or in the past put on sugar lumps to make it more palatable. The problem is that the conditions that the virus finds when it enters a human gut are just right to help it to mutate a little – just enough, indeed, to regain some of its potency. This reversion usually happens only after two to five weeks, a gap that normally allows for the person receiving the vaccine to become immune. Therefore he or she is safe from this newly-emerged "wild-type" virus. One in a million children who are vaccinated develop the disease because this mutation occurs before they have developed a successful defence.

When, however, these viruses leave the immunised person's gut they are perfectly capable of causing disease if picked up by a non-immunised person. By vaccinating large numbers of people we may be ensuring that they don't get ill, but we are also ensuring that the virus remains at large.

An alternative could be to use the Salk vaccine, in which the virus is killed and therefore carries no risk of infection. It does have two disadvantages in that it is less effective at triggering immunity in the people who receive it and the vaccine has to be injected. Switching to large-scale production of the Salk vaccine would also have its problems. The vaccine might use dead viruses, but it uses dead virulent polio viruses. Any production plant would need to be hyper-secure. That's not cheap, quick or easy to build.

The world's health managers are so sure that polio is about to be eradicated, that no-one has bothered trying to find a third option.

So, as it stands at the moment, the wild-type virus is on the retreat, but the modified virus is very much at large. While the virus can't find a home in immunised people, it can in those who have not received the vaccine. Nestling in these hosts it will take the opportunity to regain more of its virulence. Fine believes that it could take only a few years after global vaccination schemes were scaled down or stopped before there could be enough unvaccinated people to create a environmental pool of sufficient size that this new version of polio could emerge. "The question of whether OPV virus will (could, might …) persist after cessation of vaccination does not admit a simple answer," says Fine and colleague Ilona Carneiro.[4] They believe, however, that "OPV viruses could persist for several years, somewhere, in one or another population network. This may be associated with little characteristic disease and may be exceedingly difficult to detect." They stress that this conclusion is speculative, but the consequences of polio existing undercover and slowly re-establishing itself is disturbing.

Fine now believes that the only safe strategy is to continue giving the vaccine long after the last case of polio. This would buy time to think about ways of creating a new-style vaccine that can solve the problem. As Debora MacKenzie puts it in an article in *New Scientist*: "The current verdict on polio should actually be: down, but not out".[5]

And it certainly isn't out. Polio has become a prime example of how disease thrives where political trust and communication break down. In 2003, with animosity between the "Christian" West and "Muslim" East on the rise, some Islamic leaders in Nigeria started claiming that the polio vaccine contained oestrogen. This female hormone is a component of contraceptive pills and the religious leaders spread the rumour that the polio vaccine was in fact a Western plot to sterilise Islamic Africa. Soon, the vaccine was banned for twelve months until new stocks could be brought in from Indonesia, a predominantly Muslim country, and therefore one that Nigerian Muslims trusted more.

By then the mouse was out of the trap. Infection rates doubled, with over

790 children catching polio in 2004. Moreover, the resurgence of the disease allowed it to jump to previously clear countries such as Yemen, Indonesia, Ethiopia and Sudan. The official line from the WHO was that 2005 was still the target date for global eradication, but that looked highly optimistic.

In June 2005, the WHO was fighting a new outbreak of the disease in Indonesia. The first patient to contract polio in this outbreak was an eighteen-month-old child in Giri Jaya, a village in West Java. The child's symptoms of paralysis went back to early March 2005, but had only been identified as polio on May 2 that year. By May 31 a WHO mop-up team was in place and vaccinating furiously. In a three-day blitz of West Java, Banten and Jakarta, they reached 6.4 million children under the age of five. From June 28 to 29, they performed a second wave of vaccination. The costs are huge – $2.3 million just for this campaign – but the potential gain is worth it.

Monkeypox

Thankfully, there are a few signs that we are beginning to learn some of history's hard lessons, and the outbreak of monkeypox in America in the summer 2003 shows that if you stamp fast enough and hard enough on a new outbreak, you have a chance of limiting a disease's ability to spread.

When, in May 2003, three-year-old Schyan Kautzer from Dorchester, Wisconsin, had a fever, her mother, Tammy, took her to their doctor. It didn't seem a big deal, though Tammy did mention, almost in passing, that Schyan had recently been bitten by a newly purchased pet prairie dog. In recent years, prairie dogs have become popular in families, particularly in mid-western states.[6] In 2002, 10,000 of these cute looking fluffy animals were shipped out of Texas alone, to become pets.[7]

All the same, there seemed nothing to worry about. A few days later and it was a different story. Schyan's wound became discoloured, her fever was still running, and so the family set off to see the doctor again. As they left the house, they noticed that their new prairie dog was lying dead in its cage.

The doctor sent Schyan to hospital. By now she had started to get blisters on her skin and specialists scratched their heads and tried to make sense of the symptoms. Was it herpes, anthrax, plague, rabies or any one of a number of exotic possibilities? Skin specialist John Melski, who works at Marshfield Clinic, Marshfield, Wisconsin, came, took a sample of tissue from one of the blisters and sent it to a laboratory for analysis. The medics were particularly interested to examine the dead pet and sent some of its tissue for analysis. They wanted to discover what had made the rodent so unwell.

At Marshfield Clinic, infectious disease pathologist Kurt Reed ran a series of tests and called in assistance from the US Department of Agriculture and the Atlanta-based Centers for Disease Control and Prevention. Eventually they had clear results – both Schyan and her pet had caught monkeypox. She was the first person ever to have caught the disease in the USA. But by the time results were in, she wasn't alone – her parents were coming out with blisters as well. And over the next few days, reports of other cases were coming in to the Centers for Disease Control and Prevention. By the time June rolled into July, officials were taking a hard look at 80 patients who were suspected of having the disease. In one cluster alone there were 28 children who had all attended a particular day care centre in Indiana, where they had been exposed to two prairie dogs that had later died. Twelve children said they handled or petted the animals, and seven youngsters came down with monkeypox symptoms.[8]

The disease spread rapidly from state to state. On 12 June, the CDC's weekly newsletter reported suspected cases in Illinois, Indiana and Wisconsin.[9] A week later, the list included Kansas, Missouri and Ohio.[10]

Monkeypox is caused by a virus that has many similarities to that which causes smallpox, and it was first documented in 1970 in what is now the Democratic Republic of the Congo. About twelve days after being infected, the illness shows itself with fever, headache, muscle aches, backache, swollen glands and a general feeling of discomfort and exhaustion. About one to three days later, the victim develops fever and a rash of raised bumps. The first bumps normally appear on the face, but then crop up on other parts of the body. A person with monkeypox can expect to be ill for between two and four weeks. In Africa, between one and ten per cent of people who catch the disease die, but the better medical facilities in America meant that while the disease was unpleasant, there was little chance that anyone would die. You catch it from infected animals through a bite or through contact with the animal's blood, urine or any blisters that it may have. It is also possible for the monkeypox virus to be spread from person to person.

The WHO started a surveillance campaign in 1970, trying to track all individuals with the disease, and by 1986 had recorded a total of 400 cases. It didn't seem like a massive threat to health so the surveillance was turned off. After all, you can't count everything.

But when a killer virus shows up in North America, it causes a stir. It turned out that the virus had entered the USA in six giant Gambian rats that arrived on April 9: these animals are native to African rain forests. And they certainly are giant – individual animals can grow to weigh up to 5kg. These six rats were part of a shipment of some 800 small mammals that arrived in Texas from Accra in Ghana. The consignment contained nine different species – including rope squirrels, tree squirrels, Gambian giant rats, brushtail porcupines, dormice and striped mice.

One of the problems with this sort of trade is that the animals don't stay still for long. In this case, they were rapidly sent to distributors in Texas, New Jersey and Iowa. Some of the Iowa animals were further moved on to Minnesota, while others went to Illinois. The animals arriving in Illinois were again soon on their way, this time to Wisconsin, Indiana, Missouri, South Carolina, Michigan and Kansas, while a few of the Texan animals were shipped on to Japan. Before the end of April, animals from the original consignment had reached eleven states.[11]

What was needed was mass action – and quickly. By early June, state and federal officials were trying to track down the customers who had bought the animals. Pet shops were quarantining and killing the remainder of their stock of prairie dogs. Officials warned owners of these animals not to release them into the wild, but to bring them in so that they could be checked and "euthanised" if necessary.

In the second week of June 2003, the USA's Centers for Disease Control and Prevention and the Food and Drug Administration (FDA) issued a joint order banning the import of, or trade in, African rodents. This included the Gambian rats. On November 4, 2003, this joint order was replaced by an interim final rule, which maintains the prohibition on the importation of African rodents and makes it permanently illegal to sell, distribute, transport, or release these animals into the environment.

On top of this, US health authorities recommended smallpox vaccinations for anyone exposed to monkeypox. Exposure may have been either to infected pets or to people who had symptoms of the disease.[12] But vaccination is not without its dangers. To start with, estimates suggest that smallpox vaccine will only be effective at preventing monkeypox in eighty-five per cent of cases. In addition, authorities believe that a few people in every million given the vaccine are likely to die.

By stamping hard on the disease as soon as possible, officials hope that they have prevented the virus escaping into wild populations in the USA. If it did escape, it would be vastly more difficult to eradicate. By December

2003, there had been no new reports of monkeypox in the USA and it appeared the rapid clampdown had worked.

The USA had the capability to act so rapidly because of the sense of anxiety that has arisen after the September 11, 2001 attacks on New York and Washington. It goes to show that the only time to prepare for unexpected outbreaks is before they occur. This may seem expensive, particularly as the preparation should prevent a full-blown problem, and critics will therefore be able to claim that the dangers have been overplayed. History, however, shows that when you are not ahead of the disease game, you stand to lose.

"This outbreak demonstrates the importance of preparedness for the unexpected," said Tommy G. Thompson, US Secretary of Health and Human Services. "State health departments have been actively involved in planning and preparing for the possibility of a bioterrorist event. We are now seeing that this level of preparation can also assist in unexpected, natural outbreaks."[13]

The Overall Lessons

A common set of parallel threads running through all of these diseases is the way that human beings have inadvertently shaped the pattern of disease, and disease has altered human history. We'd be foolish if we believed our scientific mastery over biology was so advanced that this was no longer the case.

Three causal elements in establishing a new disease within the human population appear to be travel, starting to live in new environments and living in close proximity to each other. All three of these occur to greater and greater extents, so the possibilities of some new disease springing up get ever stronger. Pursuing leisure activities that take you into wilderness areas, or going on expeditions into rainforests, may be more adventurous than you had bargained for.

It's also worth remembering that while our greedy exploitation of the world's environment has driven many species to extinction, there is no disease-causing agent that we have completely wiped off the face of the Earth. Smallpox is the closest we have come to that achievement and let's hope the scaremongers are proved wrong and that the scientists are as good as their word at keeping this particular demon locked away.

CHAPTER 3 –
BACTERIA AND ANTIBIOTICS

Bacteria are the dominant forms of life on Earth, with more of them than any other living organism. Not bad for a form of life that exists as a single cell. Thankfully for us, the vast majority of bacteria leave us alone, preferring to live in habitats that differ significantly from the outside of our bodies or our inner workings.

There are some species of these microscopic bugs that do enjoy life inside and we welcome their presence. These include the gut-dwelling organisms that help break down food and make it accessible to us. Get rid of these bacteria by, for instance taking a course of antibiotics, and you are likely to have a bout of diarrhoea. Other bacteria live on our skin and wander around munching up any fungi that they find. Again, destroy these bugs and a fungal infection could take hold.

As is so often the case, however, it is the minority that causes trouble and gives the group a bad name. Consequently the disease-causing, or pathogenic, bacteria catch the headlines. Bacteria prove the rule that there is power in numbers, because while as individuals they are small, an infection of many millions can bring the largest of animals, such as elephants, to their knees. Or should I say flippers, as bacteria can just as easily kill the largest of animals, a blue whale.

Part of the reason why these bugs are so successful is their ability to multiply. Some are quite capable, given the right conditions, of dividing every twenty minutes. The mathematics of this are staggering. By doubling the number of bacteria at this rate you can start out with a single bacterium at six o'clock in the morning and have quarter of a million of them by noon. Six hours later you could theoretically be up to well over sixty-eight billion. This massive expansion rarely happens, because bacteria soon become overcrowded and stop growing at their full rate, but it does mean that infections can get out of hand at an alarming pace.

Naming and Blaming

It's not easy to give bacteria names. A bird watcher can sit in a hide with binoculars, getting close to the birds and using visual and behavioural clues to help make an identification. Experienced bird watchers also make use of bird calls, often identifying the presence of a bird solely on its song because the feathered friend is dashing through a dense thicket, playing hide and seek in leaf-filled trees, or is a member of a species that only comes out at night.

Microbiologists have a much smaller range of clues to help them. Scientists' initial observations were confined to staring at them down a microscope and observing their overall shape. The result of this is that most classifications of bacteria start by dividing them into three broad categories: spherical ones, called cocci; rod-shaped ones, called bacilli; and spiral-shaped ones called spirochaetes or spirilla. I've always thought that this is a bit like categorising cars based on their colour, or wine by the shape of the bottle or box in which it is contained. You might learn something, such as bright yellow cars have fewer accidents than red ones, and you never get a vintage wine in a box. But detailed breakdowns are impossible without further information.

Anyway, with thousands of different species out there, it helps to group them into catalogues, even if the rationale behind the classification is somewhat limited. The cocci group contains organisms that cause pneumonia, tonsillitis, bacterial heart disease, meningitis, a form of blood poisoning and various skin diseases. Diseases caused by bacilli include tuberculosis, whooping cough (pertussis), tetanus, typhoid fever, diphtheria, salmonellosis, shigellosis, Legionnaires' disease and botulism. The role call for spirochaetes includes syphilis, yaws, leptosporosis and Lyme disease.

Even with a microscope, pioneering microbiologists soon found that bacteria were remarkably difficult to see. The result was that they set about developing a series of chemical stains that would add colour to the bugs, but hopefully not to any surrounding material. This would make the bacteria stand out against the background.

You can imagine these early investigators dripping any dye that came to hand onto a bacteria-smeared microscope slide in a version of alchemy and looking for ways of revealing potentially valuable insights in this previously hidden world. The idea had a handy spin-off, as they soon realised that some stains worked on particular bacteria, but would not stick to others. Thus staining arrived as a second way of identifying bacteria.

One stain is worth mentioning, because we will encounter it a few times through this book. Hans Christian Joachim Gram, a Dutch bacteriologist, was working as a professor in Copenhagen when in 1884 he developed a dye that now labels almost all bacteria as either Gram-positive or Gram-negative. Gram-positive bacteria accept the dye, Gram-negative reject it.

The Gram stain involves spreading bacteria on a glass microscope slide and waving the slide in a flame from a Bunsen-burner. This makes them stick to the surface. Then the technician drips crystal violet and dilute iodine solutions on to the smear. A few moments later s/he gently washes the slide with alcohol. Gram-positive bacteria hold on to the dye and become stained a deep blue-black, while Gram-negative bacteria are left with no colour.

The reason for this difference is poorly understood. It does, however, link up with the nature of the cell wall encapsulating the bacteria. It appears that in some way the cell wall of Gram-positive bacteria hold the dye inside, preventing it from being washed away by the alcohol. Gram-negative bacteria are unable to hold the dye back.

So along with shape, the second classification is based on the nature of the cell wall. After a few years of research bacteria are now listed as either Mycoplasmas, which are surrounded by a simple membrane and no cell wall, Gram-positive bacteria, which build a single-layered cell wall, and Gram-negative bacteria, which have walls composed of at least two distinct layers.

Trying to grow the bugs can give another layer of detail. Bacteria tend to be highly specialised, thriving in exactly the right conditions but finding themselves incapable of growing if these conditions aren't met. Dropping samples of bacteria on to culture plates made to contain different nutrients will soon separate them out. Some demand small amounts of iron, others need particular vitamins or amino acids. But nutrients are not the only factor that influences growth; gases can have an affect too. Some bugs must have oxygen, others cannot exist if oxygen is present; still others are not bothered either way.

All this analysing still has only limited value and the most powerful way of identifying bacteria is to see what it does in a person. It often comes down to noting the symptoms of a disease and combining this information with a brief examination of bacteria found in a mouth swab, urine or faeces. Another approach is to take blood from the patient, extract the serum – the sticky straw-coloured fluid component of the blood – and mix it with a known strain of bacteria. If the person has been infected by this strain, his blood serum will be loaded with molecules that are tailor-made to fit on to the bugs and gather them together in clumps. So if the bacteria visibly clump together then you know the nature of the beast you are dealing with.

Causing Damage

The ideal situation for an organism is to find itself in a location where it can grow in peace and security – where nutrients are supplied to it and competitors kept away. From the point of view of some bacteria, it is therefore unfortunate that they lead to the death of their host, because in so doing they destroy their home. So what is it about bacteria that can make them so nasty?

Bacteria have two basic modes for performing their biological vandalism. Either they cause physical disruption by actually breaking into the cells of the person's body, or they sit outside and send toxic molecules that interfere with life.

Physical Assault

Loads of different bugs can establish an infection in your gut and cause dysentery – diarrhoea. For the moment we'll take a look at *Shigella*. It usually gets into people via drinking water that has been contaminated with human faeces, or on food that has been washed in this water. *Shigella* is remarkably potent. You only need to swallow a hundred or so bacteria to be in trouble, so a fly walking over your food can quite easily deliver this sort of quantity if it has previously taken a stroll on human excrement. Shaking hands with someone who has poor personal hygiene and is infected can also put you at risk.

Once swallowed, *Shigella* avoids being killed by the acid and digestive juices in the stomach and races on down to the colon. They are Gram-negative rod-shaped bacteria and once in the colon the bugs stick on to the gut wall. Genes in the bacteria then become activated and initiate the production of a protein that causes cells in the gut lining to engulf the bacteria. It appears likely that the cells that do this are the so-called M cells. The normal task of M cells is to act as the "bobby on the beat". Spotting any suspicious protein, they grab it and take it into custody. Once arrested they hand it over to cells from the immune system. These cells then decide whether it is "friend or foe" and if they don't like the look of the protein they alert the body's defensive mechanism to the element's presence. It's a biological early warning system.

When *Shigella* are captured and handed over, they don't go peacefully. Instead they burst out of the immune cell and infect normal gut lining cells.

Once in a standard gut cell they proliferate, doubling their numbers every forty minutes and breaking into neighbouring cells. From here on they leave a trail of destruction as the cells die once they have become occupied. In the layer of gut cells, the *Shigella* find themselves protected from the immune system and so grow unmolested.

Why the gut cells die is unclear, but it may simply be because the bacteria use up all of the nutrients inside the cells, leaving them no way of surviving. The consequence of this cell death is that absorption of fluid from the gut is severely reduced, hence the diarrhoea. On top of this, the damage leads to bleeding, so the stools produced are classically streaked with blood. Our intestine responds by vigorously contracting, an action that we feel as cramps. Fluid is also released in an attempt to flush any loose bacteria out of the system.

Try as they might, scientists have found it remarkably difficult to develop a vaccine that can combat *Shigella*. Either you use a form of the bacteria that is so weak that it gives poor protection, or you use a stronger one that gives nasty side effects. Antibiotics can shorten the duration of an illness, but if you give people enough clean water they will recover in any case. Giving antibiotics is controversial, because while it is nice for the individual patient to get better faster, they tend to release *Shigella* for longer in their faeces than if they had been untreated. So while they are pleased, others stand a greater chance of being infected by them. In reality, most *Shigella* infections occur in developing countries, so the rich buy themselves some drugs and gain the benefit, while, unable to afford the pills, the poor suffer the double whammy of increased risk and longer illness.

Another bug that breaks in and disturbs the peace is *Listeria monocytogenes*. In fully healthy people this is seldom a problem, at worst causing only mild flu-like symptoms. Around ten per cent of people probably have an on-going infection without even being aware of it. But in people with weakened immune systems, such as old people and those infected with HIV, the infection can be fatal.

What is unique about *L. monocytogenes* is its ability to break through to a fetus growing in the womb. The placenta normally forms an impenetrable barrier to marauding microbes, but not this one. And an infection can kill a fetus. *L. monocytogenes* enjoys hiding in processed food. Dairy products are a particular favourite, but it is quite happy to move into your home aboard foods such as fresh vegetables, shrimps, coleslaw and pâté. Pregnant women are therefore strongly advised not to eat unpasteurised products and to be particularly careful when preparing raw food.

If a food processing plant is not scrupulously careful the result can be costly, very costly. On December 22, 1998, Bil Mar Foods, a processing plant in Zeeland, Michigan, voluntarily recalled over fifteen million kilos of hot dogs and lunch meat after a listeriosis outbreak was linked to their products. Across the United States over one hundred people became ill and twenty-one died. Sara Lee, the parent company, believes that this cost them $76 million to recall the meat, and $200 million in reduced sales over the following six months.

Federal investigators believe that the contamination could have arrived attached to dust caused by work on the processing plant's air conditioning system. It was the largest meat recall in American history, and the repercussions will rumble on for years. Chicago lawyer Kenneth Moll filed a wrongful death lawsuit against Bil Mar Foods on behalf of a Tennessee man whose wife, seventy-four-year-old Helen Bodnar, died when listeria caused her to contract meningitis. Moll has also instigated a class-action lawsuit and is looking for anyone who claims to have been affected by the outbreak. On Friday May 12, 2000, Judge Jennifer Duncan-Brice gave a ruling in favour of the class-action and five individual claims. Sara Lee has agreed to pay $50,000 to anyone who ate their infected products and suffered from listeria infection for at least four days, and the company believes that the total cost will not exceed $5 million. Moll believes the figure could be as high as $100 million. While Sara Lee denies liability, The Centers for Disease Control and Prevention gave evidence that the twenty-one deaths were caused by Sara Lee's contaminated hot dogs and other meat products. Five of these cases were settled in March at a cost of $1.6 million.

The one thing, however, that we can be sure of is that as food production becomes more concentrated in a few large factories, this is the sort of crisis that we can expect to see happen again and again.

Molecular Mavericks

Other bugs don't go to all the trouble of developing ways of getting inside the body. These just establish an infection on the surface somewhere and release molecules that do the damage.

Diphtheria was one of the key causes of disease and death in infants until the 1930s. The main symptoms were a sore throat and fever. The disease is caused by Gram-positive rod-shaped bacteria called *Corynebacterium diphtheriae*, but the bacteria never gets into the body. Instead *C. diphtheriae* floats into the victim's mouth when he or she breathes and makes a home on the throat, causing a greyish film to appear. In severe infections the person's heart develops an irregular beat, they have difficulty swallowing and fall into a coma. It's quite possible that George Washington died of the disease, aged sixty-seven.

To produce these symptoms, something must be getting into the body. It's not the bacteria – they never show up in a blood sample and seem quite content to stay in the throat. The problem lies in a toxic chemical that the bacteria produce and release. It's arguably the most studied toxin, and we still have a lot to learn.

The diphtheria toxin molecule is composed of two tiny proteins, linked together by a sulphur bond. The bacteria produce it and release it into the host's bloodstream. One of the two strands of protein is shaped in such a way that it enables the toxin to gain entry into cells. Once inside, the two chains are in a more acidic environment and they split apart. The second chain then succeeds in wrecking protein synthesis within the cell, which consequently dies. It's powerful. A single molecule of toxin can kill a single cell and if that is a heart cell that the toxin entered then you are in trouble.

The disease is no longer a major problem, because at the end of the nineteenth century the Polish-born, German bacteriologist Emil von Behring discovered how to create an antitoxin. He discovered that if you injected serum obtained from an animal that had been infected by diphtheria into a second animal that had never seen the bacteria, the second animal became immune to infection. In 1901 he was awarded the first Nobel Prize for Physiology or Medicine for his efforts, and the whole world could breathe more easily – literally.

The use of this technique to prevent people from suffering when they encounter this *C. diphtheriae* has lead to an interesting situation. The vaccine given to children during the first year of their life consists of the toxin that has been treated with formaldehyde to render the protein non-toxic. Immunised people therefore tackle the toxin, rather than the bacteria. Consequently, they can continue to become infected by the bug, but they don't suffer the ill effects. This means that they can easily become walking reservoirs of disease, transporting it to places where people haven't been immunised. Deciding not to vaccinate your child therefore places him or her at risk of encountering someone who does have the disease without exhibiting symptoms.

The reason why non-immunised people in developed countries get away with it is that for some unknown reason immunisation reduces the number of toxin-producing strains of *C. diphtheriae* growing in the person's throat.

This helps to protect those in the population who have ducked out of the system.

Before you relax too much, however, you need to be aware that it doesn't stop non-toxic strains from growing. So what's the problem? The problem is that phage (a particular type of virus that specialises in living on bacteria) can move the toxin genes between strains of bacteria. One person returning from a country where the toxic strain is rife could give the bacteria to many immunised people, who have a resident population of non-toxigenic bacteria. The virus could then transfer the disease-causing genes to these resident bacteria and they in turn could then move to non-immunised people.

It seems a tall order, but some doctors think they have seen this process happening.[1] They believe that in 1977 a baby who had not been vaccinated contracted diphtheria after having been passed the bug by an older sister. The older sister, the doctors think, had a resident population of non-toxigenic bacteria that had been altered by genes from a toxigenic strain. An eight-year-old boy who had just returned from Nigeria had supposedly introduced this bug into their classroom.

So far, the only way to get at the bug itself is to take antibiotics.

Sitting Outside

Some disease-causing bacteria don't even have to come near to their victim in order to exert their evil influence. These bacteria cause disease by growing in food and releasing toxins. You can kill the bacteria by cooking the food, but you don't get rid of the toxins. Two well-known examples are botulism, caused by *Clostridium botulinum* and a food-borne disease caused by *Staphylococcus aureus*. There have been seventy-four outbreaks of botulism in the United States between 1983 and 1987 affecting some one hundred and forty people and causing ten deaths. Over the same period, *S. aureus* infections have broken out forty-seven times and made 3,141 people ill, but the bug's toxin has not killed anyone.

C. botulinum normally lives in soil or in lake sediments. Spores produced by the bacteria get on to plants growing on contaminated soil and are easily picked up by bees as they forage for pollen. The result can be spores in your honey.

Ingesting the bacteria or the spores is seldom a problem, because they can't grow well in the gut. Allowing them to grow on food and then eating the food is another story. Different varieties of the bug produce one of seven types of toxin, labelled A to G, of which type A is the most potent. The toxins work by getting into the bloodstream and being transported throughout the body. Whenever they get into the nervous system they block the action of acetylcholine. This neurotransmitter is a chemical messenger released by a nerve when it wants to pass a signal on to another nerve, or to tell muscles that it is time to contract. By inhibiting acetylcholine, the toxin paralyses the person. Once the toxin has locked on to a nerve it never lets go, so the damage is often irreversible.

The first signs start to appear four to thirty-six hours after eating the food, when the person starts to experience blurred vision and an inability to swallow or speak clearly. This can be accompanied by nausea, vomiting and headache. Not pleasant.

Botulism toxin is one of the most toxic compounds known. Ten milligrams, the equivalent of a few grains of sugar, is enough to kill twenty-five people. On a weight by weight basis, this makes it fifteen thousand times more potent than VX nerve gas and one hundred thousand times more powerful than the nerve gas Sarin, the nerve agent used in the terrorist attack in the subway system of Tokyo in March 1995. Anti-toxins exist, but the problem is always one of getting them to the patient in time.

Thankfully, *C. botulinum* hates oxygen and so can't grow on the surface of foods. The classic disease-causing situation is when food is heated, cooled and stored for long periods at room temperature. Heating drives the oxygen out of the food, and when cool the inner parts remain sufficiently free of the gas for *C. botulinum* to grow. I love bottled fruit. It's a great way of locking in the flavour of plums and blackcurrants, but it is also a great way of generating botulism if the temperatures used are too low to kill the spores. All is not lost, however, because boiling the fruit for ten to fifteen minutes before eating will destroy any toxin that may have been produced. Eating the fruit straight from the jar could be more dodgy.

Home food preserving is the main, but not sole, source of the disease. From October 15–21, 1983, some forty-five customers ordered a patty-melt from the same restaurant in Peoria, Illinois. Twenty-eight customers found that their toasted rye-bread, sliced American cheese, one-half or one-third pound hamburger and sautéed onions made them severely ill. The finger of blame pointed to the onions. Investigators found *C. botulinum* spores on onion skins that they collected from the kitchen. It appears that while the onions were prepared fresh each day, they were cooked and then kept warm in an uncovered pan and were not reheated before serving. A perfect breeding situation for these bugs. Thankfully no one died, but twelve people did need to be given help breathing when they arrived at the local hospital.

Another large outbreak in the US occurred in Michigan in 1977 when jalapeno peppers served by an Oakland County restaurant were thought to be the source of the disease. At least twenty-seven people were affected.

The UK's largest outbreak of food-borne botulism occurred in 1989, killing one person and making twenty-seven seriously unwell. They had all eaten one particular brand of hazelnut yoghurt. The bug was introduced via hazelnut purée, which had been added to the yoghurt. A small manufacturer, who made canned fruit pulps and sold them to relatively small yoghurt manufacturers, decided to diversify into making canned hazelnut paste. Sadly, the manufacturer used the same canning procedure as they always used with fruit pulps, but it proved to be insufficiently aggressive to destroy spores of *C. botulinum* hiding in the hazelnuts. Because of differences in the chemical nature of fruit pulp and hazelnuts, you need substantially different conditions to kill off the bacteria.

A New Age Dawns...

When 48-year-old London policeman Albert Alexander lay in a stinking hospital ward he was unaware that he was about to make history. Sadly, he was also not to live long enough to appreciate this.

His original injury was mild. He had a slight scratch on his face. Some say the origin of the scratch was a rose bush in his garden, others say it was a slip while shaving, but whatever the implement, it became infected. The bacteria growing in the wound must have broken out into his blood stream and started to multiply, loading the blood with toxins. He had developed septicaemia. This blood poisoning soon caused his whole face, eyes and scalp to swell. His temperature soared to 105°F.

On December 27, 1940, he entered the Briscoe Ward in Oxford's Radcliffe Infirmary. Close to death, he received massive doses of sulphonamide – the only chemical that had any hope of combating the infection – but to no effect. On February 3, 1941 the doctors removed one of his eyes and drained abscesses in an effort to combat the disease, but it marched on relentless. The infection had now reached his lung. They made a tiny puncture in his other eye to reduce pressure that was building within it and hopefully relieve some of the pain.

February 12 arrived with a new hope – literally. Dr Charles Fletcher, a clinician at the hospital, arrived in the ward with 200 milligrams of crudely purified penicillin. He injected it into the moribund policeman. Three hours later Dr Fletcher gave a second dose. Another three hours, and another dose.

Dawn rose on February 13 and the antibiotic era appeared to have been born. Already Albert's temperature was normal and he was able to sit up and eat. The relief was, however, short-lived. Within a few days all available penicillin was used. In a desperate effort to continue the therapy scientists collected Albert Alexander's urine and extracted all of the penicillin that they could find from it. But the process was inefficient and on February 19 the supply ran out. The disease became re-established and took its course. His lungs became irreversibly infected and on March 15 he died.

Although the story has been told often, it's worth repeating as a graphic reminder of the world before antibiotics. Two lessons are worth grasping. First, microbes may be microscopic, but once out of control they can kill. And secondly, a full course of antibiotics saves lives.

Chance Favours the Prepared

Victors write history. It is also recorded differently between different countries. The result is that the true story of what happened at a particular event, or the process that lead up to a "new discovery", may easily be lost in the rhetoric that surrounds claim and counter claim. No more extreme example of this can be found than the history lying behind antibiotics, where in reality a large number of people were critically involved, though popular myth only records a few, and sometimes only one.

For antibiotic discovery the names of Alexander Fleming, Ernst Chain, Howard Florey spring to mind, but you really need to add Louis Pasteur and Robert Koch. Irish mycologist C. J. La Touche shouldn't be completely forgotten, nor should the likes of Margaret Jennings, Norman Heatley and Cecil Paine.

I don't intend to give a full, blow-by-blow account of the discovery – other writers have done that time and again. But I do want to review enough of the story to help explain the science of antibiotics.

The first thing to realise is that antibiotics were discovered not invented. They have always been around in the biological world, it was a matter of realising that they were there, purifying them and making use of them. Antibiotics are chemicals produced by one micro-organism that prevents another organism from growing. In so doing, antibiotics enable an organism to create space for itself.

This was what Alexander Fleming famously spotted on a culture dish in September 1928. It appears that he had been away for a holiday in Suffolk and called into his laboratory briefly, having been asked to come into St Mary's Hospital, London, to assist a colleague who was treating a patient with a bad abscess.

Whether Fleming's attention was drawn to the top of a pile of discarded petri dishes sitting in sterilising fluid, or whether he had deliberately set up an experiment and wanted to see how it was going will be debated for ever, but the plate in question was unusual. At one edge was a mould, and on the other side of the dish were colonies of *Streptococcus* bacteria. But in a circular zone around the mould the bacteria had died – they had broken apart, or lysed as bacteriologists call the process.

Fleming had often seen mould growing on culture plates. It was a common problem of his work and he tried hard to prevent it occurring. He had also seen bacteria lyse a few years earlier, when a tear had fallen on to a petri dish. The bacterial colonies that were covered by this drip of fluid dissolved. He had even seen situations where bacteria were unable to grow next to a fungus. But he had never seen disease-causing bacteria lyse because they were near a fungal colony. This wasn't just preventing bacteria from growing, it was killing any that were present.

More than likely the mould had entered Fleming's laboratory, not through an open window but via the connecting shaft of a dumb waiter which linked his room to that of C. J. La Touche who worked in the laboratory below. La Touche was in the process of collecting fungi from all over London, in an attempt to show that they caused asthma.

In fact, it was to La Touche that Fleming turned in order to try and identify the fungus. La Touche incorrectly pronounced that it was *Penicillium rubrum*, a type of mould that we now know does not produce penicillin. The correct identity turned out to be *Penicillium notatum*. Thankfully all was not lost, however, because Fleming lodged a sample of the mould in the collection held by the Medical Research Council, so people worked away on the right mould, but just gave it the wrong name.

For the compound to be useful, Fleming realised that he needed to find a way of purifying it. Finding himself unable to do this he devoted his attention elsewhere.

This wasn't the end of the story. Antibiotics existed, so it was inevitable that they wouldn't be ignored forever. Someone was going to find a way of employing them. That task fell to Australian-born Howard Florey. In 1922, at the age of twenty-three, he had left his home in Adelaide to take up a Rhodes Scholarship in Oxford. Florey was tall, had his hair parted in the middle, wore round glasses and was a chain smoker. Colleagues described him as uncompromising, energetic and rather prickly. After excelling at Oxford, he moved to Cambridge and from there to Sheffield University. Then, aged thirty-seven, he became the Professor of Pathology at the Sir William Dunn School at Oxford.

Working with little money, Florey built up an interdisciplinary team comprised of chemists, pathologists, bacteriologists and physiologists. It was a radical concept at the time. Ernst Chain became a valuable member of the team. Chain was a chemist and set about extracting penicillin. He succeeded and injected it into a rabbit to see what would happen. If animals weren't harmed, but bacteria died, maybe this bug-killer could cure infections? The rabbit seemed unaffected.

The next thing to do was see what happened to bacteria in animals. Around this time the Oxford team had set up a Heath Robinson penicillin factory. Improvising with what was available, they used bedpans as fermentation flasks and grew *Penicillium notatum* as fast as they could.

On Saturday May 25, 1940, Chain and Florey, along with team member and biochemist Norman Heatley, performed a vital experiment. They took eight mice and injected them with 110 million *streptococci*, a virulent strain that would kill within a day. One hour later, they gave penicillin to four of the mice. The other four acted as controls and received nothing.

Heatley watched and waited. By late afternoon the four control mice were sick – they began to die after midnight. By 3.30 am all were dead. In contrast, the four treated with penicillin were fine. Heatley cycled back to his rooms through wartime, blacked-out Oxford to catch a few hours sleep before telling his supervisor, Florey.

Now they had a problem. A mouse is three thousand times smaller than a human being and their mouse experiment had used up all their stocks of penicillin. Drugs are almost always given in a dose that relates to the body mass of the recipient, because the drug spreads through the body. The bigger the animal, the more drug would be needed. To be of any use, they were going to have to scale-up the operation massively.

With the Battle of Britain in full swing, and the German Luftwaffe pounding English cities night after night, finding a way of setting up a new large-scale production system for an experimental drug was never going to be easy. In the end Florey converted a large part of the Dunn School into a factory and filled it with ceramic fermentation vessels.

Meanwhile, Heatley devised an extraction and purification system that relied on the chemical properties of penicillin. He acidified the solution containing the drug and then poured in some ether. When the two liquids were shaken the penicillin left the acidic solution and went into the ether. Most of the impurities, however, stayed in the watery acid. Stop shaking, and the two liquids separate. But now Heatley needed to get the penicillin out of the ether. This he did by shaking the ether with water that was held at a neutral pH. The penicillin came back into the clean water.

By February 1941 they thought they had enough penicillin for a human trial and gave some to poor Albert Alexander. The trial was deemed a success, even though the patient died. Again it proved the need to make more, vastly more.

Fly West, Scale Up and Lose Out

In July 1941, Florey and Heatley flew to neutral Portugal and from there they took the Pan-Am Clipper seaplane to New York. The Department of Agriculture's Northern Regional Research laboratories at Peoria, Illinois (the town that more recently was known for the botulism outbreak) gave them the biggest welcome. Heatley set to work with an American scientist A. J. Moyer.

Moyer apparently had a dislike of all things British, but put up with Heatley, though Heatley found that he became increasingly secretive. It was only after Heatley had returned to England in July 1942 that he discovered Moyer had published their work, but omitted to include Heatley's name on the publication. This subsequently allowed Moyer to patent the process with himself as the sole beneficiary. This simple move meant that all the profits from the discovery of penicillin poured into the US, with the original pioneers receiving only international recognition for their work. Fleming and Chain shared a Nobel prize in 1945, Florey was Knighted in 1944, and became Baron Florey in 1965 and Heatley received an Order of the British Empire when he retired in 1978.

Before that would happen, however, they needed to find a method of huge scale production. The laboratory in Peoria was working on agricultural waste products, growing the mould on the liquor that was left after starch was extracted from corn. Feeding Fleming's mould on this liquor helped boost the production of penicillin, but the quantities were still small.

With Pearl Harbor written into the history books in December 1941, America was thoroughly involved in the war and saw the potential for this drug. Military personnel were ordered to gather handfuls of soil from around the world and bring them to the laboratory in the hope of tracking down a fungus that naturally had a higher yield.

The might of the American Army was in the end beaten by Mary Hunt, a tea lady in the laboratory. She had earned herself the nickname of "Mouldy Mary" because of the enthusiasm with which she collected bits and pieces from rubbish bins, and one day she arrived with a decaying lump of rockmelon. The mould, *P. chrysogenum*, produced three thousand times more penicillin than Fleming's original. Problem solved. Soon American factories were making billions of units of penicillin a month and the money generated has underpinned the US pharmaceutical industry pretty well ever since. By 1979 some fifteen thousand tons of fermented bulk product were produced, having a minimum market value of $240 million, and which when purified were sold for $1,250 million.

Howard Florey and Hugh Cairns, professor of Surgery at Oxford, flew to the North African Battle Zone, taking their wonder drug with them. Antibiotic's arrival on the scene toward the end of the Second World War became a pivotal point in the history of medicine. It was also a major factor in the war. During the First World War, almost one in five of the American Army was killed by pneumonia. This fell to less than one per cent in the Second World War.

Military commanders were also impressed that one or two injections of penicillin cured gonorrhoea. As the war progressed they found themselves with thousands of troops who were incapable of fighting because of this sexually acquired disease and they were needed to form an invasion force to attack Sicily. When they asked for penicillin Florey was not keen. It appears he felt that this was an unacceptable use of his precious drug. Penicillin, he argued, shouldn't be used to salvage people who had acquired sexually transmitted diseases. General Poole referred the matter to Churchill who replied saying that "this valuable drug must on no account be wasted. It must be used to the best military advantage". Poole considered that treating these men was of great military "advantage". They got penicillin and were returned to their units.

So how has popular history left Fleming as the only name associated with penicillin? Part of the answer lies in an event in August 1942. Fleming had a friend who was dying of bacterial meningitis. He had tried for more than a week to cure him using the sulphur drugs that were all that was available. His friend was getting worse. In a panic he phoned Florey on Sunday morning asking if there was any chance of using some of his penicillin. Florey handed over all the available stock and Fleming's friend's life was saved.

So excited, Fleming announced this to the press. The wonder-drug that he had caught a glimpse of had been captured and tamed. Wearing a white coat, he had his photo taken and he sent the press to Oxford to get the rest of the story from Florey.

Florey refused to see them. He knew how short the supply of penicillin was and thought it would be immoral to raise people's hopes before they had any idea whether they would be able to conquer the problem of mass production. Fleming alone was seen in the papers and his name has been held high ever since.

History, Told from the West

Read an American book and authors seldom start the history of antibiotics with Fleming and penicillin. Instead they start a few years earlier with American soil microbiologist Selman Waksman and gramicidin. Waksman worked at the New Jersey State Agriculture Experimental Station at Rutgers University and was intrigued that while human beings excreted vast numbers of pathogenic bacteria around the world each year, one seldom found them in the soil.

Speaking in 1940 at a meeting of the National Academy of Sciences in Washington he said:

"Bacteria pathogenic to man and animals find their way to the soil, either in the excreta of the hosts or in their remains. If one considers the period for which animals and plants have existed on this planet and the great numbers of disease-producing microbes that must have thus gained entrance into the soil, one can only wonder that the soil harbors so few bacteria capable of causing infectious disease in man and animals… It was suggested that the cause of the disappearance of these disease-producing organisms in the soil is to be looked for among the soil-inhabiting microbes, antagonistic to the pathogens and bringing about their rapid destruction in the soil."[2]

His belief in the existence of soil-dwelling combatants led him and others to go soil panning, searching for the golden cure to disease. He was not disappointed. A former student of Waksman, René Dubos, moved to the Rockefeller Institute, in Albany, NY. In 1939 he isolated an antibiotic-producing soil micro-organism. The bug responsible turned out to be *Bacillus brevis*, a bacterium that excreted a substance into its surroundings that killed *Streptococcus* bacteria. Because the substance only killed Gram-positive bacteria, Dubos called it gramicidin.

It became the first naturally produced antibacterial that could treat disease. It did, however, have drawbacks. In particular, it was severely toxic when injected, but it was and still is very useful at treating surface infections.

In 1943 a second soil-originating microbe was found that had exciting properties. Another of Waksman's students isolated *Streptococcus griseus* from a chicken coop. This organism was neither a mould nor a member of the Bacillus group of bacteria. It belonged to the actinomycetes group and consequently they mixed strepto and mycete together to name the antibiotic streptomycin.

Streptomycin was a genuine breakthrough. It worked against bacteria in test tubes and it also worked in people. It killed bacteria that caused urinary tract infections, and some forms of meningitis. More exciting still, however, it could tackle *Mycobacterium tuberculosis*, the cause of tuberculosis – TB. As a drug it was far from perfect as it could cause kidney damage and deafness, but it was the first time that TB victims were ever offered a serious hope of full recovery.

I'm amused that the European excitement over penicillin normally totally eclipses this pioneering discovery. I was equally amused by a foreword to a WHO publication on the treatment of TB, written by American professor Michael Iseman, that charts the advent of antibiotics without even mentioning penicillin.[3] OK, so penicillin doesn't work against TB, but surely any history of antibiotic development really should acknowledge the story being played out on both sides of the Atlantic.

So How Do They Work?

It turns out that there are thousands of antibiotics – chemicals that are produced by one micro-organism that are capable of killing or inhibiting another. However, most of them haven't found their way on to pharmacy shelves because they also inhibit or kill people. The relatively few that are used have the fortunate property that they target a biochemical process that occurs in bacterial cells, but which doesn't occur in human cells. Ideally, the drug kills bacteria and leaves us unaffected.

Although there are now hundreds of different antibiotics on the market, scientists have managed to discover only a handful of biochemical pathways that are unique to bacteria and lay themselves open to attack. They either prevent bacteria building their cell wall, or their cell membrane, block the production of protein inside the bacterial cell, mess up the bacterium's genetic code or block specific energy handling biochemical pathways.

Penicillin strikes at the mechanism that enables bacteria to build cell walls. It blocks the cell's ability to make peptidoglycans, and without this major constituent the walls burst. This explains the lysing that Fleming first observed in his petri dish. It also means that penicillin works only on growing bacteria – because it can't take walls to pieces, it can only cause newly formed walls to be exceptionally weak. Gram-positive cells seem to be particularly susceptible, though the drug does affect Gram-negative bacteria because peptidoglycans play a small role in the structure of their cell wall.

Penicillin is now a member of a group of antibiotics that share a similar chemical structure. They all have what is known as a four-membered Beta-lactam ring as part of their make up. It is this element of their structure that enables them to act, but we will discover in the next chapter that it is also this common feature that is a weak point in their armour.

However, penicillin has no affect on the *Mycoplasma* group of bacteria, which crucially include the bug that causes tuberculosis. This is because these microbes don't have a cell wall; they are simply surrounded by a more flimsy membrane.

To combat tuberculosis you need to turn to streptomycin. This belongs to a group of antibiotics called aminoglycosides and it exerts its action by blocking the ability of bacteria to produce protein. It locks on to 70s ribosomes, intracellular units that are unique to bacteria and are critically involved in translating genetic code into chains of amino acids, the basic components of proteins. In binding to 70s ribosomes it distorts its shape and effectively throws a spanner into the works of the cell's machinery. Tetracyclines and chloramphenicols act in a similar way.

Another class of chemicals, called the macrolides, binds to 50s ribosomes and prevents the protein chain from growing. This class includes erythromycin.

A less common group of antibiotics attacks cell membranes. An example of these is polymyxin. This binds to phospholipids, the fatty component of the cell membrane. By binding, it disrupts the membrane and effectively makes it leaky. Without tight control of the flow of materials in and out of the cell, the bacterium soon dies. A problem with these drugs is that the membranes of bacterial cells are very similar to those of animal cells, so they can be dangerous to the patient and are seldom used.

Some antibiotics attack the DNA or RNA in the bacterial cell. These are the information-storing molecules that carry the bacterium's genetic code and they need to be copied each time a cell divides, so that each new cell contains a copy of the genetic sequence. One such group is called the quinolones, and an example of these is malidixic acid. This blocks topoisomerase, a part of the cellular machinery that prepares DNA so that it is ready to be copied. Once again this class of antibiotic also damages human cells and so has limited use. However, a modified version of this class of antibiotic, called the rifamycins, attack only bacterial cells and are therefore more valuable.

Chemical reactions inside cells are often enabled by proteins called enzymes. The three-dimensional structure of these molecules has pockets that are carefully shaped so that the chemicals they want to interact with can plug in. Some antibiotics exert their action by fitting into these active sites on enzymes. So called non-competitive inhibitors plug permanently into the active site and nothing can remove them. The enzyme will never work again. Competitive inhibitors move on and off the site, competing for the rights of occupation with the chemical that normally fits there. Which one wins depends on the relative concentrations of each, and if the amount of the inhibitor decreases, then the enzyme will start to work again. Isoniazide, an antibiotic used in treating TB, uses this mechanism to block a bug's ability to build mycolic acid, a vital component of the cell's structure.

The key to any antibiotic's success in treating a disease is that it kills bugs but leaves human cells unmolested.

Synthetic Suppressers

Purists claim that antibiotics are always chemicals produced by micro-organisms to fight micro-organisms. This then doesn't include any compounds that have been created by scientists. To mark the distinction, some people call these antimicrobials. In fact the quinolones that I mentioned above should strictly be classed as an antimicrobial drug rather than an antibiotic.

Sulphonamides are an important member of this group of weapons, partly because they came to the medical market just before antibiotics. Their use has largely been superseded by antibiotics, but they still play a valuable role in combating urinary infections, bronchitis, skin infections and infections of the middle ear.

Another key player in this group is Triclosan. This potent antibacterial and antifungal agent is now incorporated into products from bedding to socks, bin-liners to chopping boards and soaps to toothpastes. I looked at the ingredient list on my deodorant this morning and there it was. It is a very stable compound that isn't destroyed by sunlight, so once it is in place it stays there. It comes from the same pedigree of chemicals as the radical weed-killers 2,4,D and 2,4,5,T, the major components of Agent Orange, the defoliant that famously stripped bare the forests of Vietnam.

Triclosan brings with it the happy prospect of germ-free surfaces. Imagine the joy of a kitchen worktop that killed all bugs landing on its surface, or washing cloths that never smelt musty because the odour-generating bugs were wiped out as soon as they were wiped up.

The problem with dividing bug killers into so-called natural antibiotics and synthetic antimicrobials is that most antibiotics have at least some synthetic chemical step in their manufacture. Simple compounds like penicillin are still harvested direct from fermenting vats, but the more advanced antibiotics have been chemically altered to assist their action. Consequently, the rigid definition is breaking down and from here on in the book I will join a growing band of people who throw them all in together under a broader use of the word "antibiotic".

The Birth of a Mega-Industry

I am sure that the early pioneers would be amazed to see the legacy of their dedication and inventiveness. The scale of antibiotic production is staggering. In 1949, the United States produced over seventy-two tons of penicillin and streptomycin a year. By 1954 this had risen to two hundred tons and at the turn of the millennium the US pharmaceutical industry is pumping out a staggering two hundred thousand tons per year.

On that basis, the world should be becoming an increasingly safe place, one where our fear of bugs should be receding. But read on, because the bugs are fighting back...

CHAPTER 4 –
ENGINEERING ARMAGEDDON

There are a few moments in history where a majority of the world's population will be able to tell you where they were and what they were doing. They are triggered by events that seem to stand outside the scope of time. The 1941 bombing of Pearl Harbor; the 1963 assassination of John F. Kennedy in Dallas, Texas and the 1980 shooting of John Lennon. But none of these are etched on the fabric of collective memory with the same potency as September 11, 2001 – the day that terrorists hijacked four civilian aircraft, buried one into the Pentagon, and flew one in to each of the twin towers of the World Trade Center in New York. The fourth crashed into scrubland, possibly en-route to the White House.

President Bush announced that war had been declared on America and commentators around the globe spoke of "the day the world changed".

A more reflective voice would have probably said that it was the day the world woke up.

September 11, 2001 was certainly a shocking day, but the real terror was that the attacks came out of the blue, with no apparent warning and were witnessed live around the world. Within minutes of the first plane crashing into Tower 2, the world's media cancelled its scheduled pro-grammes to buy into the camera-shots streaming from New York. Consequently the second New York impact came live to the world. So too did the subsequent collapse of these monuments to human capitalist achievement.

We sat there in our offices and homes; we crowded around televisions in electrical shops; we witnessed the event unfold, and we learnt that a witness becomes involved in the action. Part of the power of that horrific day was that we saw it with our own eyes. We were there.

This terrorist attack was certainly the opening of a new chapter in the history of America, because while other countries have become used to terrorism in their midst, the United States of America had developed a complacency bred out of decades when warfare and mass-destruction has occurred in someone else's country. Now the US had to recognise that it too was vulnerable. Plastic coatings that had been common-place on the glass of windows in European cities for years started to be applied to panes in New York. Security systems that have been used for decades in other countries were rapidly moved into US airports.

Terrorism had come to the heart of America, but the thing that surprised many experts was the nature of the attack. While some people had previously pointed to the difficulty of defending high-rise buildings from a lunatic with a plane, most anti-terrorism gurus thought that biological or chemical agents would be the weapon of choice. Germs have an evolutionary history of success in attacking humans and many are remarkably simple to culture. A tiny pot of powder or a few infected animals could invoke mass carnage that would be extremely difficult to contain. All that is needed is an organisation that wants to create absolute terror.

A Dark History

The idea of employing germs as agents of destruction has a long history that stretches back to the fringes of recorded time and already extends into the twenty-first century.

Imagine that the year is 1348 and you are a Tartar and a member of the Mogul army. You come originally from the treeless steppes of Central Asia. Life is not desperately exciting because you are besieging Caffa, a Crimean port city tucked on the eastern side of the Black Sea that now goes by the name of Feodosija. Inside the city, the Christian Genoese seem to be surviving quite well and the siege has been going on for a couple of years. Then things get worse. Plague starts to show its ugly head in your camp and tens of thousands of your fellow Tartars die. There is no sign that this death is afflicting those inside the city. The solution is simple – share it with them – throw them some corpses.

History records that the Tartars used huge catapults to lob infected corpses of plague victims over the walls of Caffa. "The Tartars, fatigued by such a plague and pestiferous disease, stupefied and amazed, observing themselves dying without hope of health, ordered cadavers placed on their hurling machines and thrown into the city of Caffa, so that by means of these intolerable passengers the defenders died widely. Thus were projected mountains of dead, nor could the Christians hide or flee, or be freed from such disaster," reported one eyewitness.[1]

This had the desired effect. Disease spread rapidly through the city and the Genoese decided that their only option was to flee for their lives. They boarded their galleys and set sail for Italy. Despite the fact that no-one displaying signs of the disease had been allowed on board when the ships left port, only six or seven were alive on each of the twelve ships by the time they reached Messina, a port on the island of Sicily. Dead bodies littered the decks. There was a reeking smell of decaying flesh. No-one was allowed off the boats because the locals were terrified, but sadly they were unconcerned as a few rats scampered ashore. In two months, half of the inhabitants of Messina died. The plague had entered mainland Europe and the Black Death would sweep across the continent.

It's a stark object lesson in the effectiveness and danger of biological warfare. The attackers won their initial objective and shattered Caffa, but the result was far more devastating.

This wasn't the first time that disease had been used as a weapon. In the seventh century BC the Assyrians used ergot, a fungal disease of rye, to poison water supplies. Ergot produced a hallucinogen that is remarkably similar to LSD and also induces a disease that widely became known as St Anthony's Fire, so called because victims had the sensation of being burned at the stake, before their fingers, toes, hands and feet dropped off. Needless to say it makes the sufferers go berserk.

In 190 BC, at the Battle of Eurymedon, Hannibal is supposed to have won a naval victory over King Eumenes II of Pergamon by firing earthen vessels full of venomous snakes into the enemy ships, and Roman soldiers, Persians and Greeks were all reported to throw dead animals into wells to poison their enemies' water supplies.

Just to prove that it is difficult to come up with a new idea, in 1710 Russian besiegers of the city of Reval, the town now called Tallinn, used a remarkably similar tactic to the Tartars. The Russian Army had, throughout its campaign in Estonia, flung dead bodies of plague victims into the city as part of General Sheremetyev's scorched earth tactics. The general could therefore report back to the Tsar and proudly announce: "The whole country is now as bare as a desert ..."

During the French and Indian war in 1763, a British captain presented Indian officials with blankets taken from the local smallpox hospital. He reportedly said, "Out of our regard for them, we gave them two blankets and a handkerchief out of the smallpox hospital. I hope it will have the desired effect."[2] Many of the indigenous population died. Then in 1863, a Confederate surgeon tried a similar tactic, but was arrested and charged with attempting to import yellow fever-infected clothes into the northern parts of the US during the civil war.

Napoleon was never known for turning down a novel weapon and there is some evidence that when besieging the city of Mantua in 1797, during his Italian campaign, he attempted to infect the inhabitants with Swamp fever.

But, I hear some of you saying, that was history and since then we have the 1899 Hague Convention, the 1925 Geneva Protocol and the 1972 Biological Weapons Convention. None of this could happen now. Could it?

World War I saw the first violations of the Hague Convention as Germany unleashed chlorine gas against the Allies and the British, French and American forces retaliated in kind. This was despite the Convention specifically proscribing the use of poisons as weapons of war. After this war the world took stock again and in 1925 launched the Geneva Protocol, which prohibited the use of chemical and biological weapons. The US Senate, however, refused to ratify it and France only signed after making the reservation that reduced the power of the prohibition. France agreed to "no first use" of chemical or biological weapons. "The French took a you-do-it-to-us and we'll-do-it-to-you attitude," said President Emeritus of Rockefeller University Joshua Lederberg, one of the people involved in negotiating the 1972 Convention.[3] Britain and the United States followed this lead in developing a philosophy of having biological weapons as deterrents.

During World War II the Japanese operated the (secret) biological and (infamous) warfare research Unit 731 in Manchuria and deliberately exposed some three thousand Chinese prisoners to a variety of agents including plague, anthrax and syphilis. Prisoners were tied to stakes in a grid pattern and then biological weapons dropped from aircraft. The effectiveness of this was sometimes determined by live dissection of the prisoners without the use of anaesthetics. The atrocities were not confined to the Unit. At one point during the war, plague-infected rats were grown in Unit 731 and then released in China. It is believed that they may have killed at least 30,000 people in the Harbin area of China between 1946 and 1948.

It would appear that once you lose sight of the immorality of biological weapons you can lose sight of any morals. There was a huge outcry after journalist Nicholas D. Kristof published an article in the *New York Times* on March 17, 1995 that exposed this horrendous Unit. But the anger was equally aimed at the US government who Kristof claimed had agreed to a

US–Japanese cover-up. He concluded that the United States had kept its knowledge of Unit 731 a secret in return for information from the experiments, an act that in itself ignores both international law and any concept of human justice. In 2000, President Clinton pledged to release all government information on germ warfare.

If the Japanese hoped that everyone would simply forget about the Unit they were made to think again when in January, 2001 some 180 relatives of victims presented more evidence in a Tokyo court in a legal case against the Japanese government. The case is more of an irritant than any particular threat to the perpetrators as it has been running for more than four years and is not anticipated to secure any form of conviction.

During World War II the United States was involved in its own germ warfare and in 1942 formed the War Research Service. This unit looked into the possibility of using botulinum toxin and anthrax-loaded cattle cake. It appears that they stockpiled enough of these weapons so that they could be used in retaliation to any German biological attack.

At the same time the British exploded anthrax bombs on the remote Gruinard Island just off the west coast of Scotland. Sheep had been tethered to posts at known distances from the site of the blast so that weapons experts could study the extent of the weapon's effect. The island was chosen because experts said that it was so remote that the anthrax would be contained, but when cattle caught the disease on mainland Scotland immediately across the water from the fateful island, all tests were stopped. After that, humans were banned from setting foot on the island for fifty years.

Quite what was going on during the Cold War, no-one will really know, but in 1979 there was an outbreak of pulmonary anthrax in Sverdlovsk, a town in Russia's Ural Mountains. Sixty-two people died and another 259 became ill. At the time the authorities denied any link between this disease and the weapons research facility in the town, claiming that the outbreak was due to contaminated meat. Since the Iron Curtain has disappeared, they have owned up that it was due to a leak when someone forgot to turn on the filtration system and a tiny amount of anthrax-containing powder floated away in the wind.

During the outbreak, two local pathologists saved samples of brain tissue taken from victims. They hoped one day to be able to prove that the people died of anthrax from the research facility. When these were analysed in the 1990s American scientists were shocked to find not just one strain of anthrax but four different strains. It raises the possibility that the Russian researchers were deliberately creating anthrax mixtures that would evade attempts at protection through vaccination.

Who Wants Them?

Then in the 1970s the USA started pulling out of biological weapons. The reason given was that they were too unpredictable and difficult to control. As a result they were useless and the sooner they were abandoned the better. Analysts scratched their heads for a few minutes and came up with an alternative theory. Biological weapons were too good, and more frighteningly they were too simple. Once the technology was developed anyone could start to use them. The best strategy was to stop all research in the hope that this would prevent others gaining the intelligence.

With the super-power struggle between East and West gone, there was a new realisation that threats don't come in the form of massive armies and big bombs, but from small subversive organisations and so-called rogue nations. To a country or group with small resources but wanting to wage war against a stronger opponent, biological weapons could seem like an attractive concept. Deadly bacteria and viruses are plentiful. You don't have to go out of your way to find them lying around on rotten food or inhabiting soil. They are also easy to culture and grow in vast quantities. The only thing left is working out how to deliver them to their target.

Japan's Aum Shinrikyo sect showed just how easy it is to use weapons that target the biology at the centre of our being as they played with killer germs and nerve gases. It is an intriguing object lesson in how simple but also how difficult such weapons are to use in practice.

In mid-rush hour on the morning of March 20, 1995 five members of the sect joined the commuters in the underground trains. They caught trains on three of Tokyo's ten lines, the Hibiya, Marunouchi and Chiyoda lines. All the trains were due to arrive at Kasumigaseki station between 8:09 and 8:13 in the morning. On-board the trains they slid brown-paper packages under their seats, and then calmly stepped off the train. Moments later the deadly nerve gas sarin started seeping out. Pure sarin is colourless, odourless, and volatile, but commuters started to smell acetonitrile, the solvent that it was kept with. Panic broke out as passengers started gasping for breath and falling to the floor. The gas was causing their nerves to fail, thus preventing their muscles contracting. Some were sick, others lost control of their bowels and bladders. Twelve people died and 3,227 were taken to hospital; 493 were admitted. A total of over 5,500 needed medical attention. The sect members may have walked away from their deadly packages, but five years later Yasuo Hayashi, forty-two and Masato Yokoyama, thirty-five, were sentenced to death for their part in the crime. In addition, three cult members who participated in the subway gassing have been sentenced to life in prison and four more are awaiting sentencing. Five others who were indicted are awaiting trial.

While the effects were terrifying they could have been worse. It turns out that the batch of sarin they used was faulty. The group was well aware how difficult it is to use biologically active weapons because this wasn't their first attempt. In 1994 they had had a night assault on Matsumoto, a small mountain resort near Tokyo. Seven died and fifty-six people were taken to hospital as some 300 victims breathed in sarin.

The group didn't only concentrate on sarin. They had tried spraying botulism toxin from the back of a truck as it drove around Tokyo city centre and had experimented with anthrax, spraying it from the top of a tower block. Birds died, but no people.

At the time terrorism experts said that this failure to injure anyone showed just how difficult it was to use biological weapons. The assumption was that the attack failed because the perpetrators had either damaged the anthrax during preparation or that their spray had not managed to create an aerosol. In August 2001 another theory came to light. Scientists at Northern Arizona University in Flagstaff analysed samples taken from the scene of the spraying. The samples contained healthy anthrax. Clearly the sect had not damaged their germs.

These scientists then examined the DNA in the anthrax bacilli and found that it was the Sterne strain, a strain of anthrax used to generate vaccines.[4] For the people living near to the point of release this was most fortunate. This strain has been doctored so that while capable of triggering immunity, it is incapable of causing disease. This then is the most probable reason why no-one became ill. Quite why the sect used an impotent strain of the bacteria remains unclear. Maybe they were ignorant of this detail, or maybe they were just testing their systems ready for performing the real thing at a later date.

With the rise of Osama Bin Laden and the Al-Qaeda terror network to the top of the world's most-wanted list, there is now another organisation that threatens to cause alarm. Added to this allegations that Al-Qaeda had links with Iraq gave even more grounds for concern. In an August 2000 lecture, Tara O'Toole, Deputy Director of the Johns Hopkins Center for Civilian Biodefense Strategies showed a photo of the Al Hakan plant in Iraq. The plant contained fermenters brewing anthrax. It's possible to get 100,000 lethal doses in each millilitre of fluid and Iraq admitted to the United Nations Special Commission (UNSCOM) that was searching for weapons of mass destruction that it had made 8,000 litres of this lethal cocktail. O'Toole said that the inspectors suspect Iraq actually had 10 times that amount. Iraq claims that all production stopped in 1991 and that everything was destroyed when UNSCOM blew up the Al Hakam plant in June 1994. History went on to show that Iraq had probably told the truth here.

The 1995 defection of Saddam Hussein's son-in-law Hussein Kamal Hassan brought alarming details of the scale of Iraq's stockpile. Documents that he carried with him listed some 20,000 litres of botulinum toxin and 8,000 litres of anthrax spore suspension. He said that the country had also constructed SCUD missiles with a range of 300 to 600 km and capable of carrying 400-lb bombs fitted with botulinum toxin and anthrax warheads, and unmanned aircraft that were equipped with aerosol dispersal systems. It was those fears that effectively fuelled the public campaign for the assault that toppled Saddam Hussein.

There is also a continuing debate as to whether so-called Gulf War Syndrome is in fact a disease caused by an encounter with a genetically engineered bug. One theory even suggests that the causal agent may be a mutated version of HIV.

Given the shift of attention from Iraq to Afghanistan that followed the atrocity of September 11, the US government was alarmed to discover that the Red Cross run a plant in Kabul that generates anthrax vaccine. There is a strong humanitarian reason for the plant in that Afghanistan is riddled with naturally occurring anthrax, but there is also concern that the equipment that ferments the vaccine-producing strain of anthrax could be readily converted to brew up a culture of anthrax that produces the toxin.

The Poor Person's H-bomb

According to a CDC study, an intentional release of anthrax by a bio-terrorist in a major US city could result in an economic impact from $500 million to $26 billion for every 100,000 people exposed. The stakes are high. "Anthrax, sprayed from the back of an aircraft on a cool, calm midnight, could take out all of Washington DC. This could cause up to three million fatalities compared to two million from a hydrogen bomb."[5] A crank speaking? No, Graham Pearson, former Director of the UK's biological defence centre at Porton Down.

During 1998 and 1999 six thousand people across the United States were affected by hoaxes claiming that anthrax had been released. The victims spent time decontaminating areas and were given drugs to protect them should the warning be real. Imagine, suggests Joshua Lederberg, the implications for salvage and rescue if the bomb that took out the office block in Oklahoma City had had anthrax spores packed around it. The problem is that it would be too easy to do. What if one of the September 11 terrorists had placed anthrax in their checked-in baggage?

Thankfully bomb blasts or plane crashes are not good ways of disseminating bacteria or spores. They tend to travel in clumps and don't hang in the air for long. But don't relax too soon. All a terror campaign needs is some method of generating an aerosol and there are plenty of low-tech systems to choose from. An agricultural crop sprayer would be one way to discharge massive doses, though someone might spot you as you fly along – a factor that was recognised in the weeks immediately following the assault on the World Trade Center when all crop-dusters were grounded in case someone decided to "borrow" one.

There is, however, no need to get so sophisticated. Pressurised aerosol cans will do a great job, and the backpack sprayers that you can pick up at any garden equipment store will be okay, although the droplets could be a little large for ideal distribution. The best mists have droplets that are about 5 microns in diameter. But certainly if your idea is to wage a terror campaign then there is no need to set about building an intercontinental missile with a complex warhead.

When the Aum sect attacked the underground, they chose a biologically active chemical, but had they used bacteria or viruses the nature of their act would have been very different. To start with there would have been no mass panic because no-one would have been aware of any problem. A few days of calm would pass. Then one person would turn up at an emergency centre with a strange spectrum of symptoms. While the doctors and nurses were puzzling over this case another two or three similarly affected people would arrive. By the end of the day the hospital wards would be full and the authorities would be doing a good impression of headless chickens, because few cities have any well-thought-out protocol for dealing with a live biological attack. Most have plans for dealing with an explosion or a chemical spillage, and those were acted out in Oklahoma and Tokyo, but a bug would need different people doing different things.

Paramedics, fire fighters, police and specially trained rescue workers and forensic experts would be the first people on the scene of a chemical attack. Their prime objective will be to find the source and neutralise it, and then find chemical antidotes if possible. On the other hand, emergency physicians and nurses would find themselves at the sharp-end of any biological attack, with infectious disease experts, pathology laboratory specialists and epidemiologists in close support. The rush would be to identify the disease and find vaccines and suitable antibiotics.

Everyone would be looking for patterns within the disease. Are people vomiting? Do they have high temperatures? Are there any spots or rashes? Where have they been during the previous few days? All this will help the medical team establish what they are dealing with. That assumes that they are looking at a simple, single disease. To start with patients will have their own underlying infections that complicate the picture and the total collection of symptoms could be confusing if the terrorist decided to release more than one agent at a time.

From Theory to Reality

In October 2001, the world had the opportunity to see a biological attack unfold. With the dust of the World Trade Center still in New York's air, America woke-up on October 4 to a second scare. Sixty-three-year-old Robert Stevens was in hospital with pulmonary anthrax. The disease is extremely rare, and normally fatal. Stevens was an employee of American Media, a Florida-based tabloid newspaper company.

He had just returned from a three-day holiday in Northern Carolina, during which he had started to feel unwell. He had muscle ache, nausea and fever. This got worse and on October 2 his wife had taken him to the emergency department at Atlantis Medical Center. By this point he was lethargic, confused and running a fever of over 102°F (39°C). A few hours after he arrived, Stevens had a seizure. Doctors passed a tube through his mouth and into his trachea, the air passage leading to the lungs, and attached the tube to a ventilator thus enabling him to breathe. In addition they ran a high dose of antibiotics cefotaxime and vancomycin straight into his bloodstream in the hope of killing any infection. Despite this his temperature rose further.

Doctors did a thorough search for the cause of the symptoms, but found no obvious signs until a spinal tap revealed bacteria in the fluid around his brain. The hospital laboratories analysed these germs and about one day after his arrival, the hospital had preliminary results suggesting that the most likely candidate was anthrax. The health team added penicillin G to the drug regimen and started to fear the worse. His condition continued to deteriorate. Despite intense treatment, his heart started to fail and struggled to pump blood around his body. On October 4 he died.

Just as people were beginning to question this unusual event, anthrax spores were found inside the nose of another employee, Ernesto Blanco, a seventy-three-year-old Cuban-American who worked in the mail-room. It appears that he might have survived the spores because he was taking antibiotics for a chest infection.

One person with the infection is unusual – there were only eighteen recorded cases of anthrax infections in the US in the twentieth century, and they were mostly skin infections. But it can happen. Two people who work in the same building getting the same strain of anthrax that is inhaled was too exceptional to be coincidental. Still there was no direct evidence that this was a terror attack. It could be that some benign event had brought the bacterial spores into the office. The tabloid that Stevens worked on had, however, published articles that were insulting toward Bin Laden. Was this revenge?

With Blanco's illness the FBI were called in. Spores were found on Stevens' keyboard and suspicion soon fell an envelope that Blanco had delivered to Stevens' desk in the middle of September. Addressed to actress and singer Jennifer Lopez, it appeared to have come from a fan. When the letter was opened it was found to be empty except for a Star of David emblem and a folded sheet of white paper that released a fine white powder when opened. Could that have contained anthrax spores? October 10 brought a third person to the list of those identified with spores in their noses – the thirty-five-year-old woman was again an employee of the same company. Quite clearly someone had placed anthrax spores in the office in which they all worked. Although this had the hallmarks of deliberate action, it did not appear to be the actions of a well-developed bio-terrorism programme. The type of anthrax used was one that is widely available in labs around the world and is very susceptible to penicillin. If you wanted to cause real terror, you would choose one of the strains that has been engineered by people with warped minds to evade the protective capability of most antibiotics.

Early reports also suggested that this was not a weaponised sample. It's a strange term to use, but it refers to the way that the spores have been prepared. For years biowarfare designers have worked to perfect ways of freeze-drying vat-loads of anthrax-containing nutrient broth. It's a similar technique to that used to freeze-dry coffee and the idea is to remove the liquid without damaging the chemical composition of the materials. The process is used in coffee making because it preserves the flavour – in warfare it preserves the viability of the bacterial spores. The next process is to grind the resulting sludge into a fine powder. The finer the powder the more likely it is to penetrate deep into a victim's lungs.

Weapons experts initially said that the samples looked crude. They didn't have the appearance of dust particles created in a high-tech facility.

However as the weeks went by the experts started to say that this was a sophisticated batch of anthrax dust. So sophisticated that many believed that it had to have come from within the US. Part of the reason for reaching this conclusion was that the chemical cocktail surrounding the spores seemed to be made from a recipe that the US military had developed and believed was still a secret that no one else knew. This cocktail enables the anthrax dust to stay in the air for longer and float around on the wafts of air caused by someone walking past a desk, making the agent much more deadly. Given that the technique was developed by the US military, it is tempting to repeat the oft used phrase, "He who lives by the sword, dies by the sword".[6]

Still, the search was on to see if there were any signs of a link between this and September 11. Then the FBI announced that a wife of one of the editors had rented an apartment to two of the hijackers killed in the suicide attacks – could this be the missing link? Could the terrorists have posted the letter on their way to the airport?

Over the next few days panic about white powder sprang up all over the US, fuelled by fears that the perpetrators had the same disregard for human life as did the hijackers. Emergency services were stretched to the limit as countless terrified citizens called out the police to investigate numerous sightings, most of which turned out to emanate from damaged bags of flour or washing powder. But some were more sinister in that they came in otherwise empty envelopes. Was this a hoax or the real thing? Anxiety was further fuelled when an employee of a news agency in New York opened one such envelope and soon anthrax infections were showing up in the Big Apple. This was no longer a single incident – this was a campaign, but it was one that would in all probability leave many questions unanswered.

October 2001 was also a month when the authorities lost control of the public response to the incident. Thirty-eight-year-old Erin O'Connor working at NBC in New York became infected with skin anthrax after NBC offices had been sent a bug-laden letter. This obviously shook the employees, who were all given a little known antibiotic called ciprofloxacin (Cipro). That evening, NBC's news anchor Tom Brokaw held a brown bottle of tablets in front of the camera and announced to millions of viewers "In Cipro we trust".

The performance was relayed on news programmes around the world. Within days websites sprang up like mushrooms marketing the antibiotic and people flocked to their doctors to get a prescription. President George Bush became involved, threatening to remove the patent on the drug if the German-based pharmaceutical manufacturer refused to supply huge numbers of tablets at reduced cost. Two other US-based drug manufacturers joined in the fray by offering equivalent drugs free to the American public as their part of the war against global terrorism.

At this point, no one seemed to stop and ask whether pumping large quantities of this particular antibiotic into the US population was a wise idea. It was only as the number of deaths reached four and twelve others were infected that calls from antibiotic activists started to break through. By this point over 10,000 people had been prescribed Cipro and many tens of thousands were presumed to have purchased the drug and may or may not have been using it.

The problem, as we shall see in the next chapter, is that bacteria can learn to become resistant to the killing power of antibiotics. The simple rule is that the more antibiotics you pump into a system, the faster they learn.

Cipro is no different. It is one of the quinolone class of antibiotics and attacks bacteria by blocking the machinery responsible for producing copies of its genetic code. Without this equipment the cells can't reproduce and it will only be a matter of time before the bacterial infection dies out. The bacteria aren't about to take this lightly, and some of them have quirks in their machinery, which renders the antibiotic ineffective. These survive the attack and live on, passing this ability on to all future progeny. The antibiotic is now effectively useless.

Medically, Cipro is a valuable antibiotic because very few bacteria have developed resistance. It can then be used to fight infections in people where other antibiotics have failed. High volume indiscriminate usage of the antibiotic however stands the chance of producing large populations of bacteria that are resistant to Cipro, which would be a shame. Furthermore, when you take an antibiotic all the bacteria in your body perform that learning task, not just the disease-causing bugs that you wanted to attack. There may be a small population of pneumonia-causing bacteria that were previously doing no harm to you, but these may now be refined so that only the antibiotic resistant ones exist. These tougher bugs are in a strong position to set up an infection in yourself, or move on to attack some other member of the community. It could lead to outbreaks of disease far worse than the anthrax attack that was the root of the problem.

In terms of policy the dash for Cipro was all the more surprising as tests carried out on the strain of anthrax used in all the attacks soon showed that many other more commonly used antibiotics would have been equally effective. In November the health authorities started a belated attempt to curb the use of Cipro by issuing guidance that Cipro should be saved for a drug of last resort, and a more commonly used drug doxycycline used as the blanket treatment. The US health authorities recommended that penicillin should be the drug of choice for pregnant women who had been exposed to spores.

"We now have a double experiment," says Dr Stuart Levy, President of the Boston-based Alliance for the Prudent Use of Antibiotics (APUA) and one of the growing band of health experts who are anxious that the dash for this drug may have long-term consequences. A double experiment because bacteria use two different methods for developing resistance to Cipro and doxycycline. The experiment is one where scientists will be able to monitor how quickly antibiotic resistance can build up if the drugs are used incautiously. "It is a real experiment that we are going to witness on a scale that nobody could have foreseen".

Levy also pointed out that Cipro is a strange drug to employ for mass use as it has quite severe side effects. In some children, for instance, it can prevent the cartilage growing at the end of their bones and it can cause seizures. According to the experimental results recorded on the official Cipro label, adverse events that were "considered likely to be drug related" occur in 7.3 per cent of patients treated and an additional 9.2 per cent of people taking the drug have problems that are "possibly related" to the drug. A further three per cent can expect to have adverse events that are "remotely related" to the therapy. "With thousands taking [Cipro] we are not talking small numbers of people who are coming back to the doctor because they have other problems related to the medication – you can see an escalation of medical costs just on the basis of handling the side effects," comments Levy.

It wasn't just in terms of pharmaceuticals that there was clear evidence of panic driving policy. People selling gas masks had never had it so good. Most struggled to keep enough of them in stock. This was despite all the advice that a gas mask was most unlikely to help you, and may, if used incorrectly actually kill you. More than a dozen people in Israel died during the Gulf War because they used their masks incorrectly.[7] In addition, gas masks will protect you for a few hours. Then you need to change the filter canister. More problematic is the fact that you will seldom have enough warning to put the mask on. A nerve gas attack would be a sudden event, and you would only know that a germ-based attack had taken place some days later. Gas masks are only useful if there is an efficient early-warning system and then a back-up system of clean-air bunkers that you can quickly retreat to. Neither of these exist.

For weeks reports dripped in of anthrax being found in new locations, particularly around the Senate building where one of the envelopes had been opened. It pointed to one of the key problems with biological weapons, in that the spores had been transported from office to office for days before anyone became suspicious. Having the spores wafting around the postal sorting office was a guaranteed way of adding a distinct element of chaos theory to the pattern of distribution.

People bent on causing terror and others with disturbed minds are often copy-cats. They keep a look out for schemes that seem to work and then see if they can employ them in their campaign. It was not surprising that within weeks anthrax was arriving in the morning mail in countries as far from each other as Pakistan, Kenya and Argentina. Did these come from the same source, or from another? To an extent the question is immaterial. Even if these satellite attacks were the work of other organisations or disgruntled individuals, you could generate a strong argument that their inspiration lay in the initial assault. In that regard, they were all the dark progeny of the original assassin.

And what of the identity of the assassin? On November 9, the FBI introduced a marked change of tone. No longer were they looking for some member of a large international terror group. Instead they now believed it most likely that the sender of these spores was an adult male who probably had a scientific background, or at least a strong interest in science, and was waging a personal campaign against carefully selected individuals against whom he held long-standing grudges.

By mid-November some clear lessons were coming from the on-going crisis. One was that finding the source of any biological terror attack was very difficult if not impossible. As building after building in New York was closed, tested, quarantined and decontaminated, including sites of government and law, the second lesson was that containing the spread of disease is almost impossible. By the time that the first few people have symptoms, people have distributed the lethal dust on their clothes so that non-related premises become contaminated.

A third lesson was that the postal service is as good as a ballistic weapon for delivering death and disruption. This became all the more clear as two postal workers in the Brentwood sorting facility which serves

Washington DC joined the list of fatalities and the Postal Service found anthrax contamination of four of its high-speed sorting machines. This caused US postmaster general John Potter to say: "We're telling people that there is a threat – that right now, the threat is in the mail. There are no guarantees that mail is safe." The chilling concept is that, while the risk is remote, every envelope you open may have deadly bacteria inside, or may have picked up spores as it travelled through the distribution system.

Fourthly, the uneducated dash for Cipro and gas masks is a warning that no one can expect a rational response from a frightened public. All countries need regularly updated forward-planning exercises that think the unthinkable and prepare ready-made authoritative information that can be released at speed should events demand it. Without sound information, public reactions and over-reactions have the potential of transforming a crisis into a disaster.

And finally, the critical lesson must be that if you develop a weapon, be it biological, chemical or conventional, you can expect your enemy to get hold of it and turn it against you. And if ever there was a doubt, autumn 2001 taught that even used in a relatively small-scale way, bioweapons can pack a punch.

The "brilliance" of a terror campaign is that every stunt has knock-on effects for years. A small amount of anthrax released in 2001 has caused millions of dollars to be spent every year sniffing out signs of a new attack. One of the problems with surveillance systems is that the more carefully officials look, the more they seem to set off false alarms. In March 2005, the Pentagon evacuated 175 employees from a mail-handling facility after monitors had suggested anthrax was about. It turns out that this was most probably not the case, but the disruption was great. On top of this, those thought to be most at risk of catching the disease had it been present were given a course of antibiotics – just in case. There is a chance that this may ward off disease, but there is a greater chance it will stimulate resistance in all other bacteria in the area. As a consequence of the perceived threat, whole nations enter a form of group neurosis, in which policy-makers and people overreact in ways that are counter-productive.

Neighbours from Hell

America has more than its fair share of people with private agendas. When in 1984 the Rajneesh cult in The Dalles, Oregon wanted to influence the outcome of a local election they cultured a novel idea – *Salmonella typhimurium*. This they took to ten local restaurants and poured over the bowls in their salad bars. Nobody died, but 751 became ill. It took a year for police to work out what had happened.

In April 1997 Larry Wayne Harris was sentenced to 200 hours of community service and eighteen months probation. The crime was officially mail fraud: a nice catch-all law that allowed authorities to swoop on him after he had ordered three vials of plague-causing *Y. pestis* from the American Type Culture Collection in Rockville, Maryland. This is a not-for-profit company that holds the nation's largest collection of cultured diseases and ships some 130,000 cultures around the world each year. Harris had ordered the bugs using headed notepaper that gave the impression that he was a registered research laboratory. A US primetime television programme[8] claimed that the same company had supplied the Rajneesh cult with their salmonella and Iraq with a strain of anthrax known to infect humans.

Harris claims to have also tracked down the burial sites of the last animals recorded as dying from anthrax. Using a long rod, he said that he got a sample of the bug and cultured it. The real motives of his actions will probably never be known for sure, though some have suggested that his aims range from a plan to attack the New York subways, to a desire to devise cures for the disease. Whatever his background, the case serves to illustrate how easy it is to obtain lethal bugs.

The Most Likely Agents

The range of possibilities is huge, but there are some superbugs that lend themselves to the task of causing chaos. The NATO handbook dealing with potential biological weapons lists 31 infectious agents.[9] The top five are thought to be anthrax, smallpox, plague, botulism and tularemia.

Anthrax

Anthrax has always been at the top of the list of diseases that cause terror. It could even have been the causal agent in one of the first pieces of biologically aided political persuasion on record – one of the plagues that hit Egypt in the time of Moses. Ask most experts and they still count anthrax as a potent weapon. This species of bacteria (*Bacillus anthracis*) occurs throughout the world and regularly causes "natural" occurrences of the disease. Records are sketchy, but in 1958 it was estimated that between 20,000 and 100,000 people caught the disease worldwide, and the epidemic of disease that followed the accidental release of anthrax in Sverdlovsk demonstrates just how potent a weapon this could be in the hands of anyone with evil intent.

As US victims discovered, you can get infected by anthrax bacteria passing through cuts in skin, or inhaling it. Eating contaminated meat will also do the trick. Symptoms start to appear after one to five days. A skin infection kills one in five victims, while getting it in your lungs is very likely to kill you within two or three days. The bacteria release a toxin that not only attacks the victim's body, it also turns off his or her immune system, leaving them defenceless in the face of the aggressor. There is a vaccine, but it only really has any effect against the skin-acquired form of the disease. Antibiotics can help, but only if you have previously been vaccinated and then they need to be given within hours of the infection taking hold.

If you reckon you have been exposed to the bug, but have not come out with the disease then doctors will recommend a six-week course of antibiotics, either doxycycline or ciprofloxacin (Cipro). If you think you inhaled dormant spores rather than the living bug then you will need to take the drugs for longer so that you have a good level of protection as each new spore is activated.[10]

One saving grace is that anthrax is not contagious – you can't catch the disease from someone who is suffering from it. In this way any anthrax attack will be self-limiting. Once the attack has killed off the first batch of people, and the site of any anthrax release has been cleaned up, then that's the end of that episode. That said, if the spores were released from a plane flying over a populated area the clean-up operation to rid a city of spores would take years.

Scientists are hoping that they may be able to develop an antitoxin but it's certainly not going to be around for a few years. One group working at Harvard Medical School, Boston, have developed a tiny protein molecule, a peptide, that can inhibit the action of the toxin. Anthrax is so deadly because although antibiotics can kill the bacteria, if the infection has taken hold the germs will have released sufficient toxin to kill the person. Blocking the toxin is the only hope.

Anthrax toxin is released by the bacteria as three sub-units. On their own they do no harm, but linked together they are lethal. This joining up only occurs on the surface of the victim's cells. In October 2001 the Harvard team announced that their peptide could bind to one of the three sub-units effectively mopping it up and rendering the toxin inactive.[11] The peptide works well on toxins in test tubes, and early animal tests have also shown that it is effective. It will be a couple of years, however, before it could be widely available for human use.

Smallpox

Just when you thought that smallpox was dead and buried you need to think again. It could come back through a terror campaign. And it would be terrifying. Now that smallpox has been officially eradicated and all vaccination has ceased, very few people in the world have the ability to defend themselves from this killer virus. Among unprotected populations there would probably be a thirty per cent mortality rate. There is no treatment. In aerosol, viruses can survive for twenty-four hours or more and they are highly infectious at low concentrations.

For every person who had contracted the disease, there would probably be another who would be taken to hospital with similar symptoms. Two hundred victims would therefore occupy 400 bed spaces. But you couldn't just do that because they would need to be nursed in isolated wards that are kept at a reduced pressure so that air constantly flows in through cracks in windows and gaps under doors. This prevents the virus escaping. However most hospitals have very few of these specialist facilities and most are likely to be in use already, housing people with immune disorders or undergoing chemotherapy. In short the system would be overloaded.

Then 14 days later the real horror would occur as people infected through contact with the initial victims start to develop symptoms. A conservative estimate suggests that ten new cases would be sparked off by each original infection.[12] We would then have some two thousand victims and countless other panicked individuals who fortunately have some other more minor look-alike disease.

Currently there are two places where smallpox is officially held. One is the CDC in Atlanta, Georgia and the other is the Research Institute for Viral Preparations in Russia, also known as Vector. Who knows if there are any clandestine stockpiles?

On top of this, defectors from the Soviet Union have started to tell the West about work at the Russian Institute aimed at generating a newly configured smallpox virus that would be ideal for use in a warhead. It appears that by 1989 this task had been achieved and they were building dozens of tons of smallpox each year. Ken Alibek, a former first deputy chief of research for the Russian biological weapons program, has reported that smallpox viruses had been mounted in intercontinental ballistic missiles and in bombs designed for strategic use.[13] He believes they had enough biological agents to kill the entire population of the world several times.[14] Currently Vector holds 140 different strains of smallpox.

Alibek described how they had built missiles that could carry ten warheads, and inside each warhead are special bomblets filled with biological weapons. These contained cocktails of three, four or five agents. Apparently smallpox was only one of fifty-two different agents they could choose from.

The United States holds seven million doses of smallpox vaccine, just in case. But in reality the country would need 250 million doses to protect itself because the disease is so virulent that no-one in the country would be safe. And Canada would have to act quickly as well.

Once this vicious genie has been let out we might never be able to eradicate it again. Smallpox scabs saved in European labs remained effective for thirteen years so a small release could have long-term consequences. On top of this the world now has AIDS and people infected with HIV may be too unwell to cope with the vaccine so they could act as reservoirs, holding onto replicating populations of the virus.

As if this is not enough, Alibek believes that the Russians have performed a genetic marriage between smallpox and Ebola. Head of Vector, Sergei Netesov, denies this, but even the possibility that someone would think of it makes me feel sick. However a new post-Cold War fear is that Russia can no longer pay its scientists and with the borders more open they are leaving the country. Where to? Well no-one knows for certain, but according to an article in the *New York Times*, some evidence and many conspiracy theories point to Iran, Syria and North Korea.[15] With presumed reduced levels of security at the research centre, did any of these wandering scientists pack a couple of vials in their luggage?

In the summer of 2001, a few months before bio-terrorism was part of everyday conversation, a team of experts at the Johns Hopkins Center for Civilian Biodefense Strategies arranged a little exercise which for the fun of it they called Dark Winter. The key participants were all former senior government officials who acted out roles of a National Security Council. Former Senator Sam Nunn played the President.

They started by painting a scenario of an unstable political situation. The People's Republic of China had test-fired a missile that had passed through Taiwanese airspace, and an outbreak of foot-and-mouth disease in Taiwan was being attributed to deliberate Chinese action. An operative of the Al-Qaeda organisation had just been arrested in an FBI sting operation as he was attempting to buy fifty kilos of plutonium. On top of this the US had lifted sanctions on Iraq and abandoned the "no-fly" zones. Saddam Hussein had since made every effort to upgrade his military capability, and looked as if he was about to invade Kuwait. With Russian and Chinese displeasure the US is in the process of moving military hardware into the Gulf.

It's a fictitious scenario, but not completely outside the realms of possibility.

Into this global situation arrives smallpox. The announcement is made by a press officer at the White House that one person has the disease and another twenty may have it. They are all civilians in Oklahoma City. Clearly this is a deliberate attack, but quite who planted the killer germ in the heart of America is uncertain.

The exercise then attempted to simulate what would occur. Those involved had to make decisions about whether to prevent people moving from place to place and how to distribute the 12 million doses of smallpox vaccine in the US stockpile.

Dark Winter proved to be an apt title. The participants soon realised that they were completely unprepared and that there were grossly inadequate systems for coping with the situation. After eight days they had 3,000 infected people and 1,000 dead. They needed to consider whether they had the legal capability of forcing people to be vaccinated, or placing infected people in quarantine against their wish. It appeared that the "Federal Quarantine Law" did give this power, but could they get public popular approval that would enable them to carry out these restrictions in civil liberties? Dark Winter surmised that people would use their personal arsenals to fight off law-enforcement officers who came to forcibly remove infected people and take them to containment points. This would only add to the loss of life. Would the government invoke Martial Law and prohibit free assembly, ban national travel and throw whole areas of the nation into quarantine?

If they wanted it, they had one real life case of an infection breaking out in a metropolitan area that could give a little guidance as to what might happen. In 1994 plague broke out in the diamond-polishing district of Surat, on the west coast of India, just north of Bombay. Within hours of the first media reports there was panic. People fled from the city with the medical fraternity being among the first to run for their lives. With half a million people on the move the city was transformed into a ghost-town. And this was a relatively minor outbreak in which probably as few as fifty people died of the disease.

The Dark Winter simulation then looked two weeks later. By now they were facing 30,000 infected people and 10,000 dead. Smallpox had spread to twenty-five states and ten other countries. A month on and the predictions were horrific; three million with the disease, on top of one million fatalities. A letter delivered anonymously to US national newspapers demands that the US pull all of their forces out of the Gulf and Saudi Arabia, warning that if that does not happen within a week America would be hit by outbreaks of anthrax, plague and more smallpox. Contained in the letter is the genetic fingerprint of the strain of smallpox that has caused the current outbreak – clearly this is a ransom demand in a virtual kidnapping in which the mighty USA is reduced to the status of a hostage.

It might be that the world would rue the day that its scientists drew back from destroying the last stocks of this savage killer germ.

Plague

It seems that the old ones may still be the best. After thousands of years of use, plague continues to be a favourite candidate for terror. There are certainly plenty of rodents chasing around the streets and sewers of today's overcrowded cities to give the bug a piggyback into our homes and places of work were it ever to be introduced. You only need to take on-board as few as one to ten of the *Yersinia pestis* bacteria to become infected.

Plague offers the benefit of extreme simplicity for the terrorist. There is no need to have fancy timing devices that let off a lethal aerosol once you have cleared the area, indeed there is no need for a technology-based delivery system at all. Simply let the rat out of the bag.

If you wanted to get clever, the recent antibiotic-resistant version of *Y. pestis* that showed up in Madagascar could encourage you to purposely develop a drug-resistant strain. If publicity for your cause is what you are after, that would really catch the headlines.

In the 1950s and 60s, US and Soviet biological weapons programs developed techniques to aerosolise plague particles. Inhaling this would induce pneumonic plague, a particularly contagious and lethal form of the disease. The Center for Civilian Bio-defence Strategies believes that this is the likely delivery system should a contemporary terrorist decide to use it. A worst case scenario calculated by the WHO found that spraying 50kg of *Y. pestis* over a city of five million people would probably cause 150,000 cases of pneumonic plague, of whom 36,000 would be likely to die.

The first time that anyone would be aware that there had been an attack would be one to two days after release of the bacteria when there is a sudden outbreak of symptoms. There is a vaccine, but you really need to take it before being exposed to the bug. Antibiotics can help, but will have limited ability if the person has a well-established infection. Anyone who comes into contact with an infected person should start to take antibiotics for at least seven days after their last encounter with the disease.

In 2001, researchers at the Sanger Centre in Cambridge, UK, decoded the genome of the menacing *Yersinia pestis* microbe. This work showed that in its evolutionary past, this bug managed to pick up chunks of genes from bacteria that had already learnt how to infect insects, and other sets of genes from bacteria that caused human disease. Armed with these two sets of acquired knowledge, *Y. pestis* was fully equipped for its current lifestyle, partly spent in fleas, partly in mammals.

The decoding had another message. *Y. pestis* hadn't given up its quest for more genes, or its desire to sort and re-sort them within itself. Consequently, it is changing, a characteristic that makes it very hard to target either by the body's built-in defences, or by drugs given from outside. This new knowledge can be used for two purposes – either to develop ways of hitting this slippery critter, or by weapons gurus who would like to convert its resistance to treatment into a macabre asset.

Botulism

The toxin produced by botulism is the most toxic chemical known. Just 0.001 micrograms for every kilo of body weight is enough to kill, i.e. 0.075 micrograms will kill the average man. It's a speck of dust too small to see.

With botulism you have two choices. Grow the bacteria and lace people's food or water supply with it, or harvest the toxin and pump it into the air. Either could be deadly. If you can keep the victim breathing then you can keep them alive until the antitoxin arrives, in which case only one in twenty people would die. Release the toxin over crowded space, say a sports stadium, and you might not be able to get enough medical resources to enough people – the death rate could soar.

The toxin comes from *Clostridia*, a type of bacteria that grows in conditions where there is no oxygen. The disease normally occurs when the toxin is absorbed from the gut into the blood circulation. The toxin binds to receptors in the body permanently blocking the ability of nerves to trigger muscle contractions. Consequently, the person becomes paralysed. If the muscles in the rib cage become affected the person will not be able to breathe and must be ventilated. Hospital systems could cope with one or two patients at a time, but if hundreds or thousands arrived at the same time there would be no hope.

The first person would show up a few hours after an initial deliberate release of the bacteria, though the incubation time can extend for up to eight days. The initial symptoms are difficulty speaking, seeing or swallowing. The victim may well start vomiting. Recovery can take weeks or months, as the person has to develop new nerve endings to bring fresh signals to the muscles.

Tularemia

A lesser-known bug is *Francisella tularensis*, which was first discovered in Tulare County, California, in 1911. Experts consider that it is a potential bioweapon because it is highly infectious if sprayed in an aerosol. It is also one of the most infectious pathogenic bacteria known. Taking on-board as few as ten bacteria can cause the disease. Tularemia was one of the biological agents stockpiled by the US military in the late 1960s and although the US claims to have destroyed their stocks, there is no reason why other groups of people may not be fermenting supplies. Indeed the Soviet Union is believed to have continued developing drug-resistant strains of this killer right up to the early 1990s, and who knows what has happened to all those batches?

The bug breaks through the skin, the mucus membrane of the eye, lungs or gut. Symptoms of the disease include fever, chills, headache, cough and muscle pain. An estimated one in a hundred victims would die, but the rest would be ill for weeks. The 1970 WHO exercise considered the effect of releasing 50kg of *F. tularensis* over a five-million-strong metropolitan population and concluded that it would incapacitate 250,000 and kill 19,000.

Other Possibilities

The list isn't endless, but it is long enough. Cholera doesn't spread particularly well from person-to-person, but it can be caught from poorly treated water. With good medical care it shouldn't kill you, although the quip is that while languishing in bed you may wish it would.

If ever there was a nightmare scenario it would be unleashing Ebola, Marburg or any other of the growing list of haemorrhagic fevers on a city. Thankfully the killer germs would not be easy for a terrorist organisation to locate and it would be seriously dangerous for them to handle while they were culturing it and building their weapon. However, cultures of these bugs exist in laboratories throughout the world and they are always potential targets for attack or subversion. Evidence presented to a US senate committee hearing in 1995 alleged that the Aum sect have tried to obtain Ebola viruses from Zaire.[16]

And then there is always the newly realised threat of someone driving a plane into the heart of a biological research laboratory that stores killer germs. Few facilities are designed to withstand that sort of attack.

Thinking the Unthinkable

Part of the power of these weapons would be their insidious nature. Following a deliberate release, there would be a few days of calm during which any assailants could quietly slip out of the country or simply go into hiding. If the agent had been released from many sites, or worse still from a moving vehicle, then it may prove impossible to locate the source. Indeed looking for it would most probably be a waste of time.

At the end of the last millennium, the United States started to take the issue seriously. In June 1995, Clinton signed Presidential Decision Directive 39 (PDD-39) that defined the broad responsibilities and the way that different federal agencies would relate to each other in a crisis. This was followed in May 1998 by PDD-62 and PDD-63, which together started to define clear organisational structures. The aim is to have Metropolitan Medical Response Teams in each of 120 major cities, and ten specially trained National Guard units of twenty-two full-time people.

America's Central Intelligence Agency is worried. It is expecting "a tremendous increase in terrorism over the next ten years: rogue nations, terrorists, sub-national groups, cells of ethnic or religious zealots, even individuals with a grudge, are expected to attempt mass urban panic and destruction with ... widely accessible chemical and biological agents."[17] September 11, 2001 makes these words look almost prophetic.

On January 22, 1999 the *New York Times* published an interview that it had conducted with President Clinton in which he claimed that the thought of biological weapons kept him awake at night. The paper asked "how worried should we be? Is this serious today, and is the threat rising? Is it going be more serious in the future?" Clinton replied, "I would say that if the issue is how probable is it in the very near term, an American city or community would be affected, I'd say you probably shouldn't be too worried. But if the issue is, is it a near certainty that at some time in the future there will be some group, probably a terrorist group, that attempts to bring to bear either the use or the threat of a chemical or biological operation, I would say that is highly likely to happen sometime in the next few years. And therefore, I would say the appropriate response is not worry or panic, but taking this issue very seriously ... and then to try to make sure we are doing everything we can to stop this."

The only hope that nations have of being in a position to respond to a bio-weapon attack is to have a highly developed health system. One that is not permanently over-stretched with no spare capacity, and one that has built-in systems for looking out for new arrivals on the killer germ scene.

Senator Bill First says that for the USA "the number one inadequacy, if you had to rank them, is the inadequacy of our public health infrastructure – that is a product of about fifteen years of neglect."[18] It was a sentiment echoed by Dr Donald Henderson, the germ warrior who masterminded the abolition of smallpox, when he spoke to the US Senate Foreign Relations Committee on September 5, 2001. "If we do nothing more than strengthen the public health and medical care systems, we can significantly decrease the suffering and death that would follow a bioweapons attack. By being able to mitigate the consequences of such an attack, we can make ourselves less attractive targets to would-be perpetrators," he said.

Most countries have systems of disease surveillance that keep tabs on a variety of germs, but the public health officials are constantly saying that they are under-funded and over-stretched. They are not crying wolf. Working in the London School of Hygiene and Tropical Medicine, a team of disease experts looked at how well Europe was set up for detecting outbreaks of disease that occurred simultaneously in more than one country. Listing the subheadings in the results section of their report gives a flavour of their findings: "Failure to identify and report cases", "Failure to inform other countries", "Inadequate preparedness planning", "Inadequate funding arrangements", "Failure to link information to action", "Failure to provide capacity for international outbreak investigation" and "Failure to share lessons".

Despite this list, the researchers were not totally gloomy, pointing to some areas of success and improvement. A reasonable system may cope with plotting an influenza outbreak that slowly develops and spreads, but we need a good system if we are going to quash the sudden arrival of disease brought on by a terror attack. "Recognition of the nature of the event requires alert clinical services and effective reporting to national surveillance authorities. Early recognition that the event is of international importance requires swift exchange of rumour, data, and information between national authorities", say the report's authors.[19]

They don't think that a global organisation is what is needed, but do believe that there should be better sharing between nationally based set-ups. In addition, they call for rich countries to actively assist developing nations in building their disease surveillance systems, partly to help the developing nations, but also as a part of our own self-defence.

In August 2000 Tara O'Toole of the Johns Hopkins Center for Civilian Biodefense Strategies complained that there was little real effort being made to find solutions to bio-warfare. Why? Because no-one really believed it was going to happen, therefore there was no market-force to encourage people to spend time and more importantly money on that research. What was needed, she said, were faster means of diagnosing disease – waiting days for lab tests is too long. Smart vaccines and new generation antibiotics were also sorely needed. She hoped that research could uncover ways of enhancing people's immune systems so that the medical industry could get away from the "one bug – one drug" mentality that means stockpiling warehouse loads of different vaccines, each targeted against a different potential threat.

Within a couple of weeks of the World Trade Center madness, there were signs of a changing mentality with the US Biotechnology Industry Organisation circulating its members with an "urgent official request for information." The Department of Defense wanted to know what the industry could do to assist in defence against bioterrorism. As so often, it takes a shock to shake the blinkers from people's eyes.

More immediately, experts say that we need to be training our medics to spot unusual diseases. "American physicians [and to that you could add all physicians in developed countries] are not trained to diagnose illnesses due to pathogens thought to be the ones most likely to be used as bioweapons. Few physicians have ever seen cases of anthrax, or smallpox or pneumonic plague," explained Henderson.[20]

Watching planes smash into tower blocks packed with office workers brought into vivid focus that there are people in the world who will stop at nothing, literally nothing, to pursue what they feel is a righteous cause. If September 11, 2001 changes anything it should change people's attitudes. There is no room for cosy complacency that sees conflict as an issue confined to other parts of the world; that allows people to ignore the fact that we live in a global village.

CHAPTER 5 –
ANTIBIOTIC RESISTANCE

"This enquiry has been an alarming experience, which leaves us convinced that resistance to antibiotics and other anti-infective agents constitutes a major threat to public health, and ought to be recognised as such more widely than it is at present." Thus said a 1998 report of the UK's House of Lords Select Committee on Science and Technology. The comment is all the more powerful in that it comes from a body not known for issuing alarmist statements.

The World Health Organisation is also sounding positively apocalyptic: "In the last century medical advances and enhanced knowledge of the origins and causes of disease have led to an unprecedented increase in longevity and quality of life for those fortunate enough to enjoy access to drugs and vaccines. With those gifts has come a kind of complacency that could well lead humanity into the same straits as the fabled hare who slept while the turtle crept, and thereby lost the race ... Our grandparents lived during an age without antibiotics. So could many of our grandchildren. We have the means to ensure antibiotics remain effective, but we are running out of time. Our window of opportunity to help those impoverished by infectious diseases is closing."[1]

The cold reality is that only one hundred years after we realised that micro-organisms caused infectious diseases, and just fifty years after we found a terrific way of fighting them, the bugs are biting back.

The writing was on the wall as soon as antibiotics were discovered. Soon after finding penicillin, Fleming also found bacteria that learned not to be affected by the compound. He was anxious that people should be very careful when they used antibiotics. In an interview given to the *New York Times* in 1947 he warned the world that "the greatest possibility of evil in self-medication is the use of too small doses so that instead of clearing up infection, the microbes are educated to resist penicillin and a host of penicillin-fast organisms is bred out which can be passed to other individuals and from them to others until they reach someone who gets a septicaemia or a pneumonia which penicillin cannot save."[2]

It didn't help that penicillin was initially available over the counter. An August 1944 advert in *Life* magazine placed there by Schenley Laboratories, Inc, proclaimed that the weapon that saved life during the war was now "available in ever increasing quantity, at progressively lower cost". All you had to do was wander in to your local pharmacy and buy it. Given the hype that surrounded its arrival, it was taken in the misguided hope it would cure all manner of diseases. Few people knew that you needed to take a full course of treatment, and continue taking the expensive tablets to the end of the course even if the symptoms of the disease stopped within a day or two.

Resistance is seldom an all-or-nothing phenomenon. Taking antibiotics for too short a time means that you knock out the bacteria that are very susceptible, but those that have partial resistance survive to fight another day. With the easily killed bugs out of the way, these more powerful bacteria have a clean sweep of the territory and can grow faster than would have been the case if the competitors had been around. The result is that you develop your own breed of resistant disease-causing bugs that are ready to attack you in the future. In many countries around the world, antibiotics can still be bought over the counter. In this uncontrolled environment bacteria rapidly develop resistance to each antibiotic that is introduced to the market.

It wasn't just individuals that were to blame. Massive use in hospitals soon caused a crisis of its own. In 1946, just a couple of years after penicillin became available, one London hospital found that in fourteen per cent of *Staphylococci* infected patients the bacteria were resistant to penicillin. By 1950 this had increased to sixty per cent.

Streptomycin suffered a similar fate as bacteria found ways of evading the drug's attention within days of the drug being given to a single patient. This meant that the wonder treatment for TB rapidly became ineffective. It is now useful only if given with a couple of supporting agents that effectively tie-up the bug's ability to resist.

In 1973 a twelve-month-old baby went into the Naval Hospital in Bethesda with meningitis. The suspect bug was *Hemophilus influenzae*. Simple, just give ampicillin, a drug similar to penicillin. The baby died. The same thing happened a year later; this time the victim was an eighteen-month-old baby. In each case the bug had developed a resistance to the drug. Both children had been to the same day-care centre and quite possibly had acquired uniquely resistant bacteria while playing alongside the other children. Resistance had started to cause serious problems.

Gonorrhoea treatment saw a similar fate. One shot of penicillin was all that Second World War soldiers needed to get them on their feet again, but by the mid-1970s *Neisseria gonorrhoeae* became resistant to penicillin. The theory is that this resistance started in brothels in the Philippines where the women took penicillin on a regular basis to ward off the disease. Instead, they managed to educate it. Today, every country has penicillin-resistant strains of gonorrhoea doing the rounds.

Culturing Resistance

Manufactured antibiotics haven't caused resistance. They have simply expanded the amount of naturally occurring resistance. The so-called "natural world" normally operates systems of checks and balances. So it should come as no surprise that just as antibiotics are natural, so too is antibiotic resistance – antibiotic-producing micro-organisms need to have systems in place that enable them to resist their own agent of destruction.

Antibiotics have most probably been around for as long as micro-organisms have battled for their existence on the Earth – plenty of time for bacteria to learn a few tricks. It seems, however, that the bacteria that were capable of resisting antibiotic attack were never at a huge advantage over their susceptible siblings, so they never became dominant. Antibiotic resistance is probably of limited value in a natural environment because not many bacteria try to grow next to mould. So, for most bacteria, the amount of antibiotic that they are likely to encounter is very low. Also, in some cases, the antibiotic-resistant bacteria don't seem to grow as fast as their susceptible siblings, so in the absence of the agent, there is a mild advantage to not being burdened with this defensive mechanism.

All that changed in the 1940s when we learned how to produce this miracle powder. The amount of antibiotic entering some environments was huge. This was particularly the case for hospitals. Just think of yourself as an antibiotic-resistant microbe. All of a sudden you have a great advantage because you can throw up a defensive shield. While the rest of the bacterial crowd you had previously been competing with lay slaughtered, you have free access to all the available nutrients. In no time at all you are reproducing like crazy and all your progeny share your advantage. You may have been in the minority before the antibiotic assault, but now you and your sub-clan rule.

In some cases bacteria with antibiotic resistance even appear to be less virile than their non-protected relatives, but all that changes when antibiotics turn up. After all, "among the blind, the one-eyed man is king".[3]

Fleming's anxiety was that a microbe would learn how to evade the attack and pass this knowledge on to its progeny. In the age of genetic discovery we now know a lot about how that learning can occur and how it can be passed on. And the range of possibilities open to bacteria is greater than anything that Fleming feared.

The knowledge needed for biological existence is recorded in a genetic code. The code, as I am sure everyone is sick of hearing, is written using four different sub-units of deoxyribose nucleic acid (DNA). In order to grow, bacteria first enlarge and then split in two. Each new bacterium receives a complete copy of the code. Occasional errors occur during the duplicating process so that the offspring sometimes have unique abilities. Most errors cause problems and the bacterium fails to thrive, but some give that individual an advantage, and it may lead to a strain of dominant organisms.

This process is no different from the evolutionary drift that happens in any plant or animal. However, the rate at which it occurs is different. Human beings establish a new generation every twenty to thirty years. Bacteria, as we have seen, can do it every twenty to thirty minutes. In twenty years bacteria can have been through half a million generations. That is half a million occasions when that species has the opportunity of seeing the effects of a new mutation. There are also many billions of bacteria trying this random process out at any one time.

Some of these mutations have left bacteria with an ability to fight antibiotics and as expected this ability is passed to their successors. This much the early microbiologists expected. What came as a great shock was the realisation that antibiotic resistance could be handed to neighbours – not progeny, but bacteria who happened to be living nearby. The learning in one species can simply be handed over to another.

The mechanism involves plasmids, small loops of DNA that sit inside bacteria and are quite separate from the main chromosome. Yes, the chromosome mutates as it is copied and may itself contain genes that enable the bacteria to fight off antimicrobial attack – and these genes can be passed to future generations. But the plasmids are more mobile. These snippets of information can slip easily out of one bacterium and take up residence in another that happens to be in the vicinity.

The process is a sort of pseudo-sex. Two bacteria snuggle up side by side and a small tube develops between them. Rather like a sperm moving down a penis, the plasmid travels through the tube, moving safely and deliberately from one bacterium to another.

The range of abilities that plasmids can confer to a bacterium is vast. A plasmid may give a bacterium the ability to build a protein that enables it to stick to cells in the human gut lining. Another may help resist severe changes in temperature. Yet another may help give the ability to use a particular food-source, or survive without oxygen. And of course others help the owner to resist antibiotics.

Initially the solution seemed obvious. Find more antibiotics. And for a few years this seemed to be paying-off, although there were signs that all was not well. Many antibiotics appeared to attack the same biochemical pathway, so once a bacterium was resistant to one, it became resistant to that entire group. But at least there were half a dozen different classes of antibiotic available and most pundits thought it extremely unlikely that any bacteria would become resistant to more than one class.

In 1959 it became apparent that the pundits were wrong. A form of bacterial dysentery was running rife in Japan. The offending bug was *Shigella dysenteriae*. The nasty surprise in this bug was that it was resistant to four classes of antibiotic – tetracycline, sulphonamide, streptomycin and chloramphenicol. Even more shocking was the discovery that Japanese scientists also found *Escherichia coli* bacteria with an identical range of resistance. This was the moment when the scientific world realised that the genes coding for resistance must be able to gather and travel in packs. History is still being played out, but it could have been the first strike in the death-knell of antibiotics.

Remember the sixteen-year-old boy in Madagascar with the multi-resistant form of plague? Well now we can see how this happened. Prior to this case, doctors were relatively relaxed about *Y. pestis* because it had never managed to gain resistance to a wide range of antibiotics. When they studied this particular strain of bug, however, they found that the instructions giving it resistance to eight different antibiotics were all contained on one plasmid. What's more, they found that this plasmid moved easily between *Y. pestis* and the gut dwelling bacterium, *E. coli*. Sitting in people's guts, watching a vast array of antibiotics float by has enabled *E. coli* to develop resistance to a lot of different antibiotics. Most strains of *E. coli* don't do us any harm so long as their numbers don't expand too much and they stay in the lower gut. So we wash our hands after going to the toilet and don't worry about them. But the possibility of these bacteria being highly proficient at evading antibiotics and then passing this knowledge on wholesale is deeply worrying.

So, was this how the plague bacterium acquired its resistance? The answer is that we will never know for sure. In some ways it looks uncertain because for this type of transfer to occur a *Y. pestis* and an *E. coli* bacterium would have intimate contact with each other. Now, *E. coli* are normally confined to the gut, and *Y. pestis* to the lymph, spleen, liver and blood – sometimes the lungs. But the doctors who found this strain surmised that the gut bacteria could have invaded the bloodstream and met up with *Y. pestis* that way. An alternative hypothesis is that a flea could have fed on someone who had *Y. pestis* in their blood and then, perhaps, on a rat infected with a plasmid-bearing *E. coli*. The two bacteria could then have met up in the flea's gut and taken the opportunity to transfer plasmids. The newly generated superbug would then have moved into the boy when the flea bit him. Just because it might seem a little fanciful doesn't rule it out.

One thing is certain. The plasmid moved from a species of bacteria with a long history of resistance, to one that had a history of submission, and the result was a version of plague that was almost impossible to treat. "The fact that the multidrug resistant plasmid was highly transferable [in a laboratory setting] to other strains of *Y. pestis* where it was stable is of great concern," say the doctors.[4] The next time it might not respond to anything.

The fact that this bug came into existence on an island that is distant from most of the major concentrations of population in the world is no reason for complacency. Carried aboard a human host, bugs are only one plane ticket away from anywhere.

Mechanisms of Resistance

In its 1996 World Health report, the WHO said, "too few new drugs are being developed to replace those that have lost their effectiveness. In the race for supremacy, microbes are sprinting ahead."

Speaking at the American Society of Microbiology in Los Angeles in 2000, Julian Davies pointed out that resistance to penicillin was noted almost simultaneously with its discovery. Streptomycin was discovered in 1944 and used in 1947. In the same year doctors found bacteria that were resistant to it. Tetracycline was found in 1948, was put to use in 1952 and resistance showed up in 1956. You could continue the list. Every antibiotic launched has been thwarted by the rapid appearance of resistant strains.

A History of Medicine

2000 BC – Here, eat this root.

1000 AD – That root is heathen. Here, say this prayer.

1850 AD – That prayer is superstition. Here, drink this potion.

1920 AD – That potion is snake oil. Here, swallow this pill.

1945 AD – That pill is ineffective. Here, take this penicillin.

1955 AD – Oops ... bugs mutated. Here, take this tetracycline.

1960–1999 AD – Thirty-nine more "oops" ... Here, take this more powerful antibiotic.

2000 AD – The bugs have won! Here, eat this root.

Anonymous – Quoted in "Overcoming Antimicrobial Resistance" – World Health Report on Infectious Disease 2000.

So what are the tricks that microbes have learned? You can divide them into five categories: inactivating the agent; blocking entry; pumping out; altering the cellular target so that the antibiotic can't attack it; and developing a new biochemical pathway.

Inactivating the Agent

Penicillin becomes useless when bacteria learn to build an enzyme that chops it up. Cephalosporin suffers a similar fate. Scientists have now listed well over two dozen different enzymes that bugs can build, which bust these antibiotics. Part of the fight against antibiotic resistance has been to add bits to the antibiotic molecule so that it can't fit into the active site on the bacterium's antibiotic digesting enzyme and therefore evades destruction. It's no easy task modifying the antibiotic so that it is safe, but leaving it still capable of working. Any of the drugs on offer that have an "icillin" ending are modified versions of penicillin and there are plenty to choose from. However, as fast as new modifications are produced, bacteria find a way to get to them.

Rather than getting broken up, the aminoglycoside antibiotics become inactivated by enzymes adding extra units to the antibiotic molecule. This makes the molecule the wrong shape, so that it no longer performs its task. This group includes streptomycin, meomycin and kanamycin.

Blocking Entry

Some antibiotics sneak into a bacterial cell by making use of a transport mechanism designed to move molecules across the cell wall. The bacteria have the mechanism in place to pull in food, but the antibiotic looks sufficiently similar to be pulled in as well.

Penicillin slips in using this mechanism, and the first antibiotic resistance that Fleming saw in his laboratory was occurring because bacteria capable of distinguishing penicillin from their food did rather better than those who were more blasé. This mechanism of resistance is poor, however, because if you increase the concentration of penicillin it finds its way in.

Pumping Out

If the drug gets into the cell, the other way of preventing it acting is to pump it straight out again. Cell membranes are full of pumps, drawing materials in or throwing them out. It is a relatively straightforward matter to generate another pump aimed at shifting antibiotics out of the cell. Tetracycline is dealt with in this way and bacteria with the correct gene can survive in concentrations of up to one hundred times the dose used to kill naïve cells.

Cells can develop triclosan-resistance by employing similar pumps, a fact that is causing some people to have worries about the number of places that triclosan is showing up around the home. What started as a very useful agent could end up causing problems if its use is not properly controlled.

Altering the Cellular Target

Another way of rendering the antibiotic ineffective is to learn to ignore it. Bacteria generate enzymes with slightly altered shapes so that the antibiotic can no longer fit on. If the antibiotic can't latch on to the enzyme, it can't perform. Consequently, the antibiotic slips into the cell, but has no effect. Resistance to the anti-TB drug rifampin employs this system, as does resistance to quinolones.

Erythromycin exerts its bacteriocidal influence by locking on to DNA decoding ribosomes. When exposed to the drug, bacteria with ribosomes that are of a slightly different shape avoid this insult and continue to grow.

Developing a New Biochemical Pathway

The final trick up bacteria's sleeves is to side-step the antibiotic completely. The resistance gene goes one step further than just modifying the old enzyme. This time it provides the code needed to build a completely new enzyme that performs the function blocked by the antibiotic. This is the method employed to evade the wiles of sulphonamides and trimethoprim.

And Now for My Next Trick

If bacteria merely stuck to developing resistance to the antibiotics that they had seen, things would be a lot simpler. Instead they have another cunning tactic. It's so powerful it looks like magic, because growing bacteria in the presence of a single antibiotic produces a colony that is resistant to many antibiotics.

One study looked at women who were taking the antibiotic tetracycline to cure urinary infections. They took the drug for many weeks and as they swallowed tablets, the antibiotic flowed throughout their bodies. Soon *E. coli* in the women's guts started to appear with resistance to tetracycline. Then they showed up with resistance to other antibiotics. Some became resistant to at least six other agents. Bacteria colonising the women's skin also followed a similar pattern. All it takes is a couple of weeks of a single antibiotic for bacteria to become inventive.

So how do they do it? One theory was that the multi-resistant bacteria were present and in selecting for plasmids with tetracycline resistance, you just happened to pull in plasmids that also had resistance to other antibiotics. A nice theory, but antibiotic campaigner Stuart Levy describes how his research team at Tufts University School of Medicine, Boston, produced startling evidence. They found that bacteria could perform the same tricks in the controlled environment of a clean laboratory test tube. They started with a strain of bacteria with no resistance to antibiotics and no plasmids, and kept them in test tubes with small amounts of tetracycline. Soon they developed resistance to seven different antibiotics. Some of these antibiotics were synthetic ones that have never been seen in a natural environment. It is as if they are building defence mechanisms against zones of weakness just in case an adversary should choose that line of attack.

But, I ask again, how do they do it? No-one knows. The main message though is that they can. Taking one antibiotic can be all it takes to trigger multidrug resistance. It strikes me that it is worth making sure that you really need them before you swallow them.

Helping the Foe

Taking antibiotics can make you more susceptible to bacterial disease. A 1981 outbreak of salmonellosis was traced back to a brand of pre-cooked roast beef in New Jersey. About one hundred people became ill. The surprising finding was that people taking antibiotics at the time of the outbreak were more likely to be attacked by the *Salmonella* than non-users.

The rationale for this is easy to follow. Taking antibiotics clears out disease-causing bacteria and normal bacteria in a person's gut. This leaves an empty territory that is waiting to be colonised by new bacteria. If food-borne bacteria come along that are resistant to the type of antibiotic being taken, then they have a wonderful time. There is no competition and numbers expand like crazy. Of course if the *Salmonella* was susceptible to the antibiotic then this wouldn't happen, but *Salmonella* – like all bacteria – are learning.

Tuberculosis – A Case History of Resistance

I have more than a passing interest in antibiotic therapy for tuberculosis (TB). It's arguable that without streptomycin I wouldn't be here.

My father caught TB shortly after the end of the Second World War. In the spring of 1947 he was studying at St David's University in Lampeter, Wales, and had recently seen Jean, one of his sisters, die of the disease. Jean lived on the family farm in North Wales, and he had cycled back to college. He loved college life and with fitness developed from a childhood working on a farm and a recent period with the army, he was one of the front-runners in the cross-country team.

Knowing how fit he was, he was unconcerned when all the students were told to attend a mass chest X-ray. "I remember sitting in the college dining hall, looking around and thinking, I wonder which of these poor people have TB?" he explained. "I never thought that it would include me. The X-ray showed shadows on my lungs. Still, streptomycin had come out, so they gave me the drug – the worst of it was that I wasn't allowed to do any more cross-country."

No symptoms developed so he assumed that the disease had gone away. After Lampeter he moved to Oak Hill theological college just north of London, and three years later took his first job as a trainee parish priest in Illugan, Cornwall. In the spring of 1954 he went down with 'flu. He recovered, but when talking to his doctor decided to have another chest X-ray, just to check that all was clear. It wasn't. The medics decided that more radical treatment was needed. Clearly the streptomycin hadn't cleared the disease, and the bacteria were now probably drug-resistant.

Although he still never suffered the symptoms of the disease, surgeons in the nearby Tehidy Hospital performed a heroic operation to remove a large section of one lung and some of the other. The legacy of this is a huge scar across his back that stretches from his hip to his shoulder, giving the impression that he has at some point encountered a shark. He was put on the new regimen of streptomycin and PAS (Para-amino salt of salicylic acid). "I particularly remember the PAS, because it was a huge tablet." This was post-war Britain – the "make do and mend" generation. One of his hobbies was marquetry, making pictures using thin slices of different coloured wood, which required a fine hobby knife that he was constantly sharpening. Armed with this skill for precision sharpening, it wasn't too long before he took on the task of sharpening the hospital's hypodermic needles.

By 1955 he was well enough to move to the Edward Bolitho Convalescent Home, an isolation unit built on a hill above Newlyn Harbour. Slowly, over his six-month stay, his strength returned. Along with helping him recover, the time in hospital was supposed to keep him away from the rest of the population so that he couldn't spread the disease. "I found it almost unbearable sitting day after day in the grounds looking down on the beach and watching people swim in the sea," he told me. As he recovered, however, he and a couple of other patients took to jumping out of their window in the wooden hut that served as their bed-room and taking nocturnal walks along the sea front.

He survived to tell the tale, and was one of the last to have surgery to excise infected lung tissue, because with the new wonder drugs at hand that dangerous operation was no longer needed.

TB was no joke. In the 1800s it killed about one per cent of the population in some cities. While the incidence of disease in developed countries saw a sharp decline from the 1950s this pattern was not followed elsewhere. As the new millennium dawned, some two billion people were believed to be infected, with a further eight million new cases being recorded each year, making TB one of the most common infectious diseases worldwide. Two million people die of it each year. In developing countries, TB causes six per cent of all infant deaths and one in five adult deaths. What's gone wrong?

At almost the same time that Waksman's student Albert Schatz came upon streptomycin, Jorgen Lehmann, a scientist working in Gothenburg, Sweden, synthesised para-amino salt of salicylic acid (PAS).[5]

This turned out to be another chemical that could attack TB bacteria. Within years it became apparent that using either treatment alone bred drug-resistant organisms faster than it got rid of the bugs. So came the notion of using the two together. This improved the situation, but bacteria still managed to become resistant.

Then, in 1952, three different groups of scientists came upon isonicotinic acid hydrazide (INH) – then and now the single most effective treatment against *Mycobacterium tuberculosis*. With a third string to their bow, doctors felt more confident. Triple therapy could cure all but the most severely ill, so long as it was given properly. Sadly, not everyone adhered to recommendations and so the numbers of drug-resistant bacteria continued to increase.

To an extent, people were relaxed about the arrival of resistance. As far as the scientists could tell the drug-resistant bacteria were much less capable of causing disease, so they weren't much of a threat. Consequently most of the anti-TB programmes in Europe and the United States were wound down and funds directed to what appeared to be more pressing needs.

That was until HIV entered the world map. HIV's main activity leads to victims' immune systems being blown apart. They become susceptible to all sorts of infections, especially TB, and the drug resistant strains of TB find them easy prey. Now HIV infection and subsequent AIDS is running hand-in-hand with TB in the vulnerable populations of Africa, Europe and the United States.

As HIV marches into Asia, TB is running rife. India bears the unfortunate accolade of being the country with the highest number of cases in the world, with more than one thousand people dying of it every day. Countries like Bangladesh, Cambodia, China, Indonesia, Pakistan, the Philippines, Thailand and Vietnam are among the leading nations for infection rates. In some areas TB is crippling the economy as children have to leave school early to look after dying parents. UNICEF's Kul Gautam says that, in many cases, having the disease causes you to be cast out of your family. Many women land up being ostracised by their families and communities, which in turn has a devastating impact on the well-being of their children, families and society in general. Speaking in Hyderabad, India, on World TB day 2000, US President Bill Clinton pointed out that "These are human tragedies, economic calamities, and far more than crises for you, they are crises for the world. The spread of disease is the one global problem from which… no nation is immune."

Antibiotic resistance in TB demonstrates how easily multidrug resistance can be acquired literally against the odds. Natural resistance to drugs arrives by mutation as bacterial DNA is copied when bacterial populations grow. By watching how often this occurs, scientists have worked out the probability of this event for each antibiotic. In the case of INH, one in every one thousand million (10^8) bacteria spontaneously acquires resistance. The odds of this happening are remote but, as we have seen, populations of bacteria do a lot of growing, so it does happen. Similarly, streptomycin resistance occurs in one in every one thousand million bacteria.

To calculate the probability of both forms of resistance occurring spontaneously in a single bacterium is easy. Just multiply the two figures together. The result tells us that only one in every ten thousand million million (10^{16}) bacteria would achieve this. Now this really is unlikely.

But what if you only give patients one of the drugs and then some time later start with the other? In this case you could generate a population of bacteria that were resistant to the first drug. When these bacteria meet the second agent we are back to needing only a 10^8 event to achieve resistance to this new drug. Thus it's relatively easy to increase incrementally the numbers of antibiotic resistant genes. WHO figures show that almost half of people with TB in Nepal have bacteria resistant to two or more antibiotics. About one third of those in New York City and one eighth in Bolivia and Korea suffer from multidrug resistant bugs. In Europe, multidrug resistance has been found in France, England, Wales and Germany.ᵒ Nowhere seems to be exempt. The WHO reports multidrug resistance in one third of new cases of TB in Estonia and in almost half of patients in the Slovak Republic who had received at least one previous course of treatment. A 1997 WHO report found drug-resistant TB-causing bacteria in thirty-five countries from five continents.

Tuberculosis control campaigns around the world have been poorly coordinated. In some countries patients are simply given tablets and sent on their way. If the people are poor they may choose to take some and sell others, or may share them around their family in the mistaken belief that it will help everyone. Instead, it means that no-one is getting a proper dose and the bacteria love it. Other countries are starting to employ a DOT system – Directly Observed Therapy. This requires patients to come to the clinic on a regular basis and swallow the tablet before leaving.

Disease thrives on disorder, and TB has certainly gained ground in Eastern Europe, reversing the previous century of decline. The chaos caused as the socialist health system crumbled has been accompanied by an increase in the death toll from TB in Russia and the countries of the former USSR.

Poor and cramped housing conditions make great breeding grounds for TB, and prisons can be hothouses of infection. The numbers of people in prison around the world are difficult to determine precisely, but ten million is a good estimate and about ten times that number pass through prisons and detention centres each year. Prisons are not populated with a representative sample of the community. Instead they are loaded predominantly with men aged fifteen to forty, who belong to minority groups and come from poor socio-economic groupings. Compared to the average member of the population, these people are at increased risk of getting the disease in the first place, and packing them together in small, overcrowded cells simply serves to exacerbate the situation.

A prison in California in 1991 that housed 5,421 inmates and employed fifteen hundred staff suddenly found that they had eighteen cases of active TB. Not a massive epidemic, but a rate that is ten times higher than in the general population. Furthermore, ten of the people, including one member of staff, acquired the infection in the prison. On top of this another 324 showed signs of having been exposed to the infection, but had mounted a successful immune response and fought the bug off.

In 1999 the International Centre for Prison Studies, based at King's College, London, published a report that summed up the situation in its title "Sentenced to Die? – The problems of TB in Prisons in Eastern Europe and Central Asia". It pointed out that in the countries of the former Soviet Union the situation is dire. In the Russian Federation, for example, estimates suggest that one hundred thousand prisoners have active TB – ten per cent of the total prison population. Of these, some twelve thousand have multidrug resistant strains of the bug. In another report, journalist Angela Charlton describes conditions at a prison in Tula, 110 miles south of Moscow. The prison contains ten thousand prisoners. Ninety people pack into cells that were initially designed for thirty, and even with the correct number of inmates it would have been tight. Malnutrition is the order of the day and the idea of prisoners' rights is yet to penetrate post-glasnost Russia. It comes as no surprise to find that more than fifteen hundred of the men have TB. Ten miles down the road, a thousand-bed facility houses convicts, every one coughing and wheezing with TB. The conditions are less cramped, but more hopeless. Few are being cured.

There is no room for complacency in the community outside the prison. At the very least authorities need to consider that as people are released at the end of their sentence, they bring the bugs with them. Thirteen thousand Russian prisoners with TB are freed in an average year. With a failing health system there is little hope for appropriate treatment.

The United Nations Standard Minimum Rules for the Treatment of Prisoners makes some laudable statements. It requires that no individual should bring TB into a prison, that no prisoner should be exposed to TB while in prison, and that no former prisoner should take TB back into the community. They are nice ideals, but almost impossible to uphold. Health policy-makers need to take the issue seriously, however, because there is no way that you will be able to control TB adequately within a country unless you control it inside prisons.

Finding ways of protecting communities from TB has taxed our skills and imaginations. Between 1770 and 1892 on the east coast of North America the belief spread that TB was caused by vampires – recently dead people who return at night to feed on the blood of the living. Exhuming the suspected vampire and examining the body was the first step toward stopping these clusters of disease. Quite often suspicion would fall on someone who had themselves died of TB. Blood in the heart or signs that the body was decaying at an unusually slow rate were taken as proof, and the body's head would be removed and placed on the upper chest. The heart was removed and burned.[7]

Vaccination holds out more hope and doctors have given over three billion doses of BCG vaccine. This consists of a non-virulent strain of M. bovis named after French bacteriologists Léon Calmette and Camille Guérin, the co-discoverers of BCG (Bacillus of Calmette and Guérin). It is cheap to make and the lack of toxic side-effects make it one of the safest vaccines in the world, but it has limitations. It is reasonably good at preventing children from getting the disease, but does not protect adults. Also, it is no good if the person already has a pre-existing TB infection.

With the numbers of people getting the disease increasing, more attention is being given to building a new super-vaccine, but there is nothing in the pipeline that stands a good chance of preventing people getting TB in the first place. Consequently, effective antibiotics that can combat disease will remain a vital part of our armoury for the foreseeable future.

This makes it even more important that health policies work to keep resistance at bay. Once plasmids exist with the knowledge to resist antibiotics, they can spread rapidly through bacterial populations, and as we saw with plague, there is no particular reason why they should remain in the type of bacteria in which they originated. The spread of a strain of TB bacterium that is resistant to all current treatments could turn back the clock to the pre-antibiotic era, the time when TB was incurable. Not a nice thought.

From MSRA to VSRA

Another difficult bug to control is Staphylococcus aureus, a species of bacteria that made early surgical operations distinctly hazardous. While the discovery in the 1840s, by Charles Jackson, that ether is an anaesthetic opened the possibility of performing surgery, patients were suddenly introduced to new sources of infection. *S. aureus* lives on the skin and takes any opportunity to cling to a knife and dive inside during surgery. Once there it is a short step to a lethal infection.

Surgery only started to become safe after Joseph Lister introduced the idea of asepsis – working in a bug free zone. Penicillin was a thrilling development and it worked wonders – for about eighteen months. But then the *S. aureus* learned how to chop it up. Methicillin came along in 1959 and again the bug looked beaten. Once more *S. aureus* fought back and *Methicillin Resistant S. aureus*, known as MRSA, was on the scene. While this is unfortunate it's not a total tragedy because we had vancomycin, another antibiotic that seemed invincible.

In 1999 doctors moved a sixty-three-year-old woman from a long-term care facility to a hospital in Illinois, USA. She was seriously unwell, with advanced kidney disease and tubes entering a number of veins. She had MRSA and so was given vancomycin. This failed to stop bacteria growing in her blood and after just over a week doctors found that she had bacteria that were resistant to this drug. Ten days later she died. This was the fourth recorded case of disease caused by vancomycin-resistant bacteria in the United States. Vancomycin resistance is slowly becoming more common with reported sightings in Japan and Scotland.

At the moment these vancomycin-resistant bacteria are fairly rare. But that is no reason for complacency, and is no consolation if you happen to be the person who they decide to inhabit.

Life on Deadly Surfaces

Resistance seems to know no bounds. Disinfectants are a group of nasty chemicals that rip bacteria to pieces. They are not normally classed as antibiotics because they don't disrupt a specific chemical process within bacteria. On the whole they are also not used in medical treatments, because they are likely to damage the patient.

Triclosan is an interesting variant on this theme. Until recently it was thought of as a disinfectant, killing a wide range of Gram-positive and Gram-negative bacteria. As it is a stable chemical it has found its way into many products. As a chemical that is tolerated on our skins, it has even got into deodorants, soaps and toothpastes.

Because people thought that it wasn't an antibiotic, they thought that there was no issue with resistance. But now that is under debate. A 1998 paper written by Laura McMurry and colleagues at Tufts University School of Medicine, Boston, USA, and published in the science journal *Nature*[8] found evidence that triclosan blocks a specific pathway. In other words, it was acting as an antibiotic, and moreover they found that resistant bugs were emerging.

This sheds new light on triclosan, and probably some other disinfectants. Until this discovery there were few worries about indiscriminate use of these chemicals, but if they are antibiotics, they could start to trigger resistance, and that is more worrying. The researchers found that triclosan seems to work by messing up a bacterium's ability to build fatty components of their cell membranes. If this is the case, its action is similar to drugs used to combat *E. coli* and *M. tuberculosis*, so resistance to triclosan could potentially engender resistance to these life-saving drugs.

A result of this is that commentators like Stuart Levy say that we should use antibiotic-containing soaps and ointments to clean wounds, but use normal soap and warm water on all other occasions. This is likely to conserve the effectiveness of these powerful chemicals.

In a Class of Its Own

April 2000 saw Zyvox enter the fray. This is a new weapon and belongs to the first new class of antibiotics to be launched in thirty-five years. It attacks a new biochemical pathway affected by no other antibiotics. The American Food and Drugs Administration (FDA) gave the go-ahead for its use against certain skin infections, pneumonia and serious infections that follow surgery. It works by blocking the bacteria's ability to build proteins.

Its makers, Pharmacia & Upjohn Inc, are thrilled and believe that it will be invaluable in fighting multi-resistant bacteria. They also believe that because it is a totally synthetic compound bacteria will find it difficult to generate resistance to it. However, even while trials were running there were reports of resistant strains in three patients.

This leads to an interesting debate in the best way to make use of this valuable drug. Pharmacia & Upjohn would love to see it used as a first-choice antibiotic. According to financial analyst Jack Lamberton, who works with HSBC Securities, this could generate sales of $1 billion per year. On the other hand, commentators such as Trish Perl, an infection control officer at the Johns Hopkins Hospital in Baltimore, claim that this could also accelerate bacteria's acquisition of resistance to Zyvox, and therefore hope that it will be reserved for use as a drug of last resort.

Zyvox comes hard on the heels of Synercid, another new antibiotic this time produced by Rhone-Poulenc Rorer. It's composed of two compounds, quinupristin and dalforpristin. However, unlike Zyvox's novel mode of action, Synercid works in a way that is similar to other antibiotics. Add to this the fact that it has been used for a number of years in European animal feed and we have the distinct possibility that bugs have had time to work out mechanisms of resistance.

Farming Resistance

All our efforts at slowing down the acquisition of resistance and developing new antibiotics could be thwarted if we don't get antibiotics under control on the farm. "Of the six billion animals raised for human consumption in the United States yearly, most receive antibiotics during their lifetimes. In any one year, domestic food animals outnumber humans in the United States by more than five to one," states Stuart Levy. Globally about a half of the antibiotics manufactured are fed to animals. It's a multi-billion dollar business and manufacturers are reluctant to see the market taken away. The consequence of feeding antibiotics to farm animals is, unfortunately, that these beasts provide a superb environment for bacteria to learn how to resist antibiotics. That resistance can then bolster human disease.

Farmers give antibiotics to their animals for three reasons. One is to treat disease. The second, which is more contentious, is to prevent animals picking up diseases in the first place. And the third, which is highly contentious, is to promote growth. The British Veterinary Association claims that "Antimicrobal use has contributed to improved food safety standards, by reducing the likelihood of meat, egg and milk products presenting disease problems for the consumer or those concerned with their production. In addition, freedom for animals to receive treatment for disease is incorporated in the Welfare Codes and therefore is justifiable on welfare grounds."[9] The association points out that antibiotics should be given after the disease has been accurately diagnosed and ideally tests done to check that the bug is sensitive to the antibiotic of choice. One problem, however, is that the farmer is very likely to want to start a course of therapy before the test results are known. In addition, they say that wherever possible veterinarians should prescribe narrow spectrum drugs, which are less likely to cause large-scale resistance.

Few people disagree with using antibiotics to treat disease. But the quantities used can, however, be huge because the animals are large. A cow can weigh ten times as much as a human and will need ten times the dose to achieve a similar effect. Farm animals also produce huge quantities of bacteria-laden faeces and if they are being fed antibiotics, these bacteria must be resistant to the drug in order to have survived. A typical human bowel movement throws out one hundred million, million, million bacteria. Cows produce up to five hundred times the volume of faeces as do humans. Do the calculation. It's a lot of resistant bacteria landing in the environment.

Preventive uses of antibiotics also need the drugs to be given at high therapeutic doses. The drug is added either to feed or water and is used to prevent outbreaks of disease that a farmer predicts could easily occur. "This is the situation where the antibiotics are used to compensate poor management or extreme intensification of production," says Henrik Wegener, a Danish research professor linked to the WHO. For example, some intensive agricultural systems are so poor or stressful for the animals that disease is highly likely to occur if preventive medication is not given. "A sophisticated example is when American pig producers medicate piglets in order to be able to remove them from their mothers as early as two weeks of age," he explains. This is called "medicated early weaning" and the purpose is to have the sow back in production as quickly as possible. Piglets at that age are very fragile, partly because their immune systems are not fully matured. Removed from their mothers, they can survive only with the support of antibiotics. Antibiotics are used in these systems of "factory farming" to overcome barriers for increased productivity defined by the animals' natural biology.

No-one knows why feeding animals small amounts of antibiotics can increase their rate of growth, but in the 1950s the practice started and now some seven million kilograms of antibiotics are fed to US farm animals each year. Experiments to see how the antibiotic was having its effects showed that you got no growth promotion in animals born and bred in sterile environments. The point of interest is that these animals had no on-board bacteria. The conclusion is that the drug must be working through some influence on bacterial populations.

At first sight, the dose used seems to be too small to wipe the bacteria out, but as many antimicrobials pass through the gut unmetabolised they become more concentrated. This is because ninety per cent of the food matter is absorbed. As a result the concentration in the lower sections of the animal's gut and in its faeces may be five or ten times higher than it was in the feed. Wegener believes that the concentration of the antibiotic avoparcin toward the end of a chicken's gut is twice the concentration needed to kill susceptible bacteria. This is also the area of the gut where the bacterial load is at its highest. This potential source of resistance is also alarming because the nearest human medication to avoparcin is vancomycin – our antibiotic of last resort.

Another consequence of antibiotics passing through the animal is that farmers are slowly filling the soil with antibiotics, and that can encourage growth of resistance in bacteria that exist outside the animals. In February 2000 European Union officials caused a stir when they relaxed the rules about how much antibiotic is allowed to accumulate in farm soil. Previously the limit had been 7.5 g per hectare, but the limit was raised to 75 g – a ten-fold increase. Remarkably, in changing this regulation the EU paid little or no attention to the possibility that it could influence the development of antibiotic resistance in soil microbes.

In 1997 the WHO sent out a press release entitled "Antibiotic use in food-producing animals must be curtailed to prevent increased resistance in humans". A meeting of seventy health experts on October 17 that year had concluded that there was clear evidence that resistant strains of *Salmonella, Campylobacter, Enterococci* and *E. coli* had been transmitted from animals to humans. The meeting recommended that the use of any antimicrobial agent for growth promotion should be terminated if it is used in human medicine or known to select for cross-resistance to antimicrobials used in human medicine. Furthermore, it is recommended to have a systematic approach towards replacing the use of antimicrobials for growth promotion with safer non-antimicrobial alternatives.

Fluoroquinolone use was highlighted for particular concern. In Europe there is now a ban on feeding any antibiotic that is currently used in medicine for the purpose of promoting an animal's growth. The hope is to prevent a build-up of resistance to life-saving drugs. We've seen earlier that even this degree of caution may have limited benefit as giving one antibiotic can induce a whole raft of resistance. There is, however, no restriction on using any class of antibiotic for combating disease, whether in the form of therapeutic use or preventative use.

In the US at the moment there is less caution, though the FDA is starting to look at the situation. In 1998 it published "A Proposed Framework for Evaluating and Assuring the Human Safety of the Microbial Effects of Antimicrobial New Animal Drugs Intended for Use in Food-Producing Animals (Framework document)". This has launched a procedure that is about as long and convoluted as its title, but the aim is to collect evidence to see whether there is definite proof of danger. It's going to take years before the process is concluded. "Our rationale is that we are becoming increasingly concerned about the emergence of food-borne bacteria that may become resistant to antibiotics that are necessary in the treatment of those food-borne diseases in humans," said Stephen Sundlof, director of the Center for Veterinary Medicine at the FDA.[10]

The US pharmaceutical and agricultural industries on the whole think that the issue is getting blown out of all proportion. "We're not saying there isn't any concern," says Richard Carnevale of the Animal Health Institute, which represents US animal-drug producers, "but in the whole scheme of things, we believe that it's relatively minor." The producers believe that inappropriate prescribing to humans is causing the majority of antibiotic resistance.

Denmark has taken the opposite approach. Through the mid- to late-1990s they introduced a voluntary ban on the use of antibiotics as growth promoters. Rapidly they saw a massive reduction in the number of resistant bacteria around the farms. For example, in 1995 more than three-quarters of *Enterococcus faecium*, a bacterium that can cause human disease found on poultry farms, were resistant to vancomycin. By 1999 this had reduced to one in ten.[11]

The big surprise in Denmark was that they saw no reduction in the animals' rate of growth when the so-called growth promoting antibiotics were withdrawn. In fact, in poultry production, the animals' average weight at forty-two days went up from 1,960 g to 2,000 g. The chicken ate fractionally more food to get to this weight than animals fed antibiotics, but the savings made by not putting the expensive drug into the food more than paid for the additional consumption. "This reduced cost was surprising to us and to the producers, as we all expected that it would have some consequences in terms of reduced slaughter weight, or increase feed requirement," says Wegener. "My personal opinion is that growth promoters are not promoting growth in modern, highly advanced animal production systems, but they may serve as prophylaxis for certain types of disease."[12] As evidence for this he points to a small increase in the amount of antibiotics used to treat disease in Danish flocks – from 2 kg to 24 kg – which occurred in 1998. This was needed to compensate for the removal of 1,500 kg of antibiotics that had been used as growth promoters in the previous year. "The pharmaceutical industry is fighting very hard to maintain their market. I hope that they have seen the writing on the wall. I even believe they have. But they are trying to buy time, and I can understand that they are wanting to do that for commercial reasons. So what we can argue about is not if the use of growth promoters should be phased out, but how fast."

Wegener also believes that it if we are not careful dollars rather than clinical need can influence veterinary prescribing of antibiotics to clear up infections on farms. Speaking at the 100th Annual Meeting of the American Society for Microbiology, he presented evidence that limiting the profit that veterinarians can make from ordering antibiotics massively reduces the amount of antibiotic they prescribe. His evidence comes from data tabulated by The European Medicines Agency, which shows the way that antibiotic use varies in different countries. He compared this to the quantities of meat produced. Using this information, Wegener calculated the average quantity of antibiotic used to produce one kilogram of meat.

His estimates reveal a six- to seven-fold variation in the use of therapeutic antibiotics between different European countries. The UK, Greece and Spain use 100–150 mg of antibiotics per kilogram of meat produced, while countries like Ireland, Sweden and Denmark use less than 25 mg/kg. According to Wegener, "These differences cannot be explained by any single agricultural factor." Wegener believes that clues to the cause can be found in a recent report from the UK[13], which estimated that forty per cent of the income of veterinarians came from the sale of drugs. The UK report stressed that there is "no evidence that UK veterinarians are abusing prescribing practices in order to maximise revenue from the sale of drugs. Indeed, it would be unethical for them to do so". Wegener is sceptical. "This is a very strong incitement to write a prescription," he says. "It suggests that a veterinarian would not visit a client without giving a prescription. Otherwise he cannot make a decent living. At best it may colour his opinion." In fact, the report acknowledged that without this income "some veterinary practices would not survive."

Evidence in Denmark shows that restricting the profit that can be made by selling antibiotics reduces their use. In 1995, rules were introduced preventing veterinarians making more than a five per cent profit on the sale of these drugs. By 1996, the use of therapeutic antibiotics had fallen by forty per cent. Wegener points out that you can't prove the link, but it looks suspicious.

In his book *The Antibiotic Paradox*, Levy recounts plenty of examples showing that we need to be worried about farm-bred antibiotic resistance. He points to a 1983 outbreak of *Salmonella Newport* in four Midwestern states that were traced back to a single South Dakota farm. The problem was that the bugs had developed multi-resistance on the farm, and this hampered clinical attempts to clear up the disease in humans. A similar outbreak in 1985 affected several hundred Californians. Two died. This time the CDC traced the bugs back to a farm where the cattle had been fed therapeutic and sub-therapeutic levels of antibiotics. "This was the first definitive study, using biochemical and microbiological techniques, that traced the causative micro-organism from an animal source to humans via all parts of the food chain," comments Levy.[14]

He also documents how quickly farm workers and their families can be affected. During the 1970s his laboratory started feeding oxytetracycline to newly hatched chicks on a farm in Sherborn, Massachusetts. Another group of chickens on the farm received no antibiotics. The farmer's family lived in a house about two hundred feet away from the chicken shed. Within 24-36 hours of starting to eat the antibiotic, the bacteria in the chicks' guts had developed resistance to it. After five to six months, the same thing happened in the guts of the farm family members.

A German study showed that resistance can break out of the farm. Pigs fed growth-promoting levels of streptothricin, a previously unused antibiotic, had resistant bacteria within six months. Within two years, resistant bacteria were found in one in six *E. coli* taken from farm workers. Not only that, but it showed up in people who happened to live in the area. In addition, streptothricin-resistant bacteria were found in one per cent of people who lived nearby who had urine infections.

The question is, how long will it be, and what sort of crisis will it take, before we take the issue seriously?

Are Antibiotics Dead?

Antibiotics are still incredibly valuable drugs. Most diseases still respond to at least one class of them, and there is no doubt that day by day they save lives, reduce the duration of a disease and protect vulnerable people from infection. It is because of their power that we need to treat them with respect so that we have them in the future.

No-one wants to return to a pre-antibiotic era when a scratch could kill, but some people who are not known for making wild statements are starting to suggest that could happen. They are beginning to sound scary. In the year 2000, George Poste, former head of research at SmithKline Beecham, gave a grave warning. "There will be a radical change of public perception from around 2002 onwards. People will get a sore throat on Tuesday and be dead by Friday. It's going to be a rude shock to society."[15] The increase in antibiotic resistance as we move into the twenty-first century shows that the general idea is well-founded.

Levy backs up this sentiment. "Given what we are seeing already, it is not difficult to envision a total microbial change in favour of resistant forms. Under these circumstances, unless humans developed a solid immunity to bacteria, we would face a dreaded time when our ability to treat infections would be doomed to failure. The world might seem like a replay of the uncontrollable plagues of the Dark Ages."16

One of the problems is the time taken to create, test and launch a new drug. While bacteria develop new strategies in hours and days, drug companies can take up to fifteen years to research a compound, test it in animals, run small trials in human subjects and perform more wide-spread clinical tests. The time needed is to satisfy our desire for safety. Penicillin went from isolation to full-scale production and marketing in a couple of years. Current regulatory frameworks ensure that that pace could never happen again. Thalidomide taught us that we need to be careful with new entries to the pharmaceutical market, because after all we don't want to cause more harm than good.

Let's Be Sensible – and Quickly

The USA's Alliance for the Prudent Use of Antibiotics (AUPA) claims that about a third of the one hundred and fifty million antibiotic prescriptions written each year in the USA are inappropriate. One study found that as many as seventy per cent of patients with colds and viral sore throats were given antibiotics. Director of Antimicrobial Resistance for the CDC, Dr Richard Besser, told an audience of physicians attending a medical conference that in his opinion each year US physicians write $50 million worth of prescriptions that are ineffectual and unnecessary. Looking at it another way, the CDC has also estimated that fifty million of the one hundred and fifty million outpatient prescriptions written in the USA for antibiotics each year are unneeded.

It's mad. And it's dangerous. There is a desperate need to get away from the mindset that says, "Oh, take antibiotics just in case. It can't do any harm and might do some good". The plain truth is that it could do some harm, both to the individual taking the drug and to the community who then suffer from an increased chance of resistant bugs floating around.

There is a clear trail of blame. Scientists are blaming doctors and doctors blaming patients. The patient walks in feeling unwell. She is anxious about missing time from work and is keen to get a quick fix. The solution is obvious – or so it appears: a prescription for antibiotics. The problem is that most colds, bouts of 'flu and sore throats are not caused by bacteria, but by viruses. Let's say it again. Antibiotics can't touch viruses. In fact, by disturbing the bacterial population, they stand a chance of making a viral illness worse.

Some patients are difficult to persuade and all too often doctors use the prescription pad as a way of ending an appointment so that they can get on with the rest of their list. It's difficult to blame them; the patient is sitting there demanding antibiotics and threatening to go elsewhere if they are not handed over.

The body is also remarkably good at fighting most infections unaided. It just takes a few days to achieve this. This time delay gives the false impression that antibiotics are the real saviours. Let's look at a standard time course. Your two-year old child has been crying and pulling at his ears for a couple of days. He is obviously feeling lousy. You go to the doctor and are given some antibiotics. It's a sticky banana-flavoured syrup that dribbles off the spoon and is sprayed over your clothes as you push the spoon into the child's mouth. But a good deal is swallowed. Three days later the child is better. Hooray for antibiotics! Well, maybe not. Unless your child has a particular problem, there is every chance that the child's own immune system would have fought off the bug in more or less the same amount of time without the antibiotic. In fact, unknown to you, the child was quite possibly on the way to recovery by the time the doctor signed the prescription.

Some observers go as far as saying that as few as one per cent of prescriptions are actually needed. We need to develop a mentality that realises that taking an antibiotic is a social decision. In the short term it might help or hinder your health. In the long term it is likely to contribute to a reduction in the drug's overall effectiveness.

Patients need to stop asking for antibiotics as if they were some magic cure-all, and the medical technologists need to develop cheap, rapid test systems that would allow a doctor to take a throat swab and look for bacteria before prescribing a jar of pills. At the same time doctors need to spend more time educating their patients about the power of antibiotics when they are used correctly and the limitations of antibiotics when misused. This way we may preserve the effectiveness of our current armoury for long enough to see new drugs come on stream.

CHAPTER 6 -
BIRD FLU: A VAGRANT VIRUS

As the trial of Saddam Hussein started in mid October 2005, the West's media was divided about what to put on its front pages – a man accused of killing tens of thousands in the past, or a disease that could kill tens of millions in the future. Avian Influenza, or bird 'flu for short, had just arrived in Europe. To make sense of the catastrophic predictions of what may happen we need to look at another agent of destruction, and look at what viruses have done in the past. And viruses are curious objects.

If it's difficult to deal with bacteria because they learn how to resist being killed, how do you cope with disease-causing agents that were never alive in the first place? Enter the world of the virus. These particles of biology are difficult to classify because they are more than a complex chemical but less than a living organism – less even than a microscopic organism like a bacterium.

At its most basic, a virus is simply a particle of biological material that can form copies of itself. You could argue that that would serve as a definition of many bacteria, but the difference is that viruses cannot duplicate themselves on their own. Put a virus in a solution of nutrients and nothing happens. They need the assistance of living cells. A virus is simply a short sequence of genetic code wrapped in a protein package. It has no cellular machinery that would enable it to do anything with that code. Essentially, it has none of the ribosomes needed for producing proteins, nor the mitochondria needed for handling energy.

Viruses are quite capable of existing in the environment for months and years, effectively dormant. They can hide away undetected and unnoticed, waiting for the right combination of events to trigger their re-emergence. To multiply, however, they must gain entry into a cell. Some have preferences for plant cells, others for animals. Some, the bacteriophage, thrive on bacteria.

The first stage in understanding the disease-causing nature of any viral particle is to find out why it targets any particular cell type. The answer lies in the unique protein molecules that each strain of virus uses to build its coat. These proteins allow it to grab hold of specific receptors on the surface of specific cells and, once contact has been established, they have a variety of ways of breaking in. Like a house guest from Hell, they take control of the cell, re-ordering priorities so that the cell's machinery becomes devoted to serving the virus.

All energies are now focused on building new viruses. Within hours if not minutes, this normal cell can become packed with virulent particles. The cell becomes the unwitting host to a viral orgy. In many cases the host cells then burst, releasing the viruses, all the cell contents and metabolic wastes. You can often tell if a virus has infected your cells because your temperature would suddenly rise as the particles erupt into your blood stream. In fact, some viruses take such a regular time from infecting cells, through duplication and on to release, that they cause a predictable pulsing fever, with the person's temperature soaring each time particles burst forth. Each peak of fever marks another generation in that branch of the viral kingdom.

Where viruses have appeared from is open to debate. Some scientists maintain that they have arrived from space aboard meteors and are evidence of life-forms in other parts of the Universe. Others suggest that they could have evolved from bacteria that have found that they can exist quite happily, thank you, without all the encumbrance of sub-cellular factories. For my part, I'm not going to get anxious about where they came from, the important thing is that they are here and capable of wreaking havoc.

The Legacy of 1918

If you are ever in doubt about the destructive capability of viruses, just mention 1918 to a medical historian. "Spanish Influenza" will be the immediate response. The First World War was drawing to a close, a bloody conflict that had claimed the lives of nine million people. The world was reeling. Worse was to come, this time not in the shape of bullets, bayonets, blast bombs and nerve gas, but a simple virus. Young people would wake up feeling fit and healthy, but be dead by the evening. They had a viral 'flu, dubbed Spanish 'flu not because it originated in Spain, but because Spain was hardest hit – one in four of Spain's population was affected, a high ratio even for this brutish bug. Around the world an estimated two billion were infected. Where it came from we will never know for sure, and possibly more worryingly, we don't know where it went because in 1920 it disappeared without trace.

This wasn't the sort of illness that causes people to phone in sick and then be back at their desks within a couple of days. That's normally just a heavy cold and it confuses the issue to call it 'flu. Real 'flu is serious. Victims started by complaining of fevers and sore throats, but soon felt as if they had been beaten all over with a club. Autopsies of Spanish 'flu victims revealed swollen, wet lungs filled with enormous quantities of thin, bloody fluid. The tiny air pockets that normally allow oxygen to get into blood – and carbon dioxide to leave it – were full of fluid. The passages leading to the throat were filled with a bloody froth of fluid and air. In many victims doctors found clear signs of bacterial infections that had taken advantage of the lung damage and set up shop. Without enough oxygen, the sufferers became cyanotic; in other words they turned blue. The discoloration started at the ears and spread all over the face. When people died the lung fluid would often flood out and drench the bed sheets. One unusual feature of this 'flu is that it seemed to prefer to attack young people – most take out the elderly.

The first reported case was on March 4, 1918, in Camp Fuston, in Kansas, when a single person reported sick. A week later, on March 11, an army private went to his medical team at Fort Riley, Kansas. By lunch time Fort Riley had one hundred in the sick room – by the end of the week they had five hundred seriously ill solders, and forty-eight had died.

The 'flu's rapid progress around the world was aided by the war effort as one and a half million American soldiers crossed the Atlantic to support the final stages of the war. Many of them caught the virus while crossing, and some never made it to Europe. Those who did introduced it to an unsuspecting continent.

Even so this first wave of the disease was mild – that is in relation to the version of the disease that emerged in the autumn. This second wave had all the appearance of being the same virus, in that anyone who had caught the spring virus and survived was immune, but as the virus wallowed in the battlefield mud it had mutated and was more nasty. August 22 in Brest, France, and the new variant of this agent reared its ugly head. Within days it showed up in Boston and Freetown, Sierra Leone, carried there aboard US and British military vessels. The virus paid no respect to boundaries or treaties. It entered Portugal and then attacked Spain, infecting eight million of its population. From there it crossed the Pyrenees and went on into France, moving on to Italy and England. Scandinavia caught it from England and Sicily caught it from Italy. European and American ships gave it free passage to Iceland and American ships took it to New Zealand. Spanish 'flu arrived in India by sea and travelled inland aboard the railways.

In a matter of months it swept around the world and killed at least twenty million people – some commentators put the death toll at forty million. That's in the order of one per cent of the world's population at that point and at least twice the number killed by the war. The United States contributed half a million to the death toll – twenty thousand died in New York alone; 7,600 died in Philadelphia within a fourteen-day period. Entire communities in remote areas of Alaska were wiped out. One in twenty of Ghana's population died in September and October 1918. In November and December thirty-eight thousand residents of Western Samoa became infected by the virus, 7,500 of whom died. Thirty-five thousand people died in Sweden. I could go on.

With such carnage, facts and myth rapidly merge. There were reports of a woman boarding the subway in Coney Island just outside New York feeling mildly ill, and being found dead when the train arrived forty minutes later in Columbus Circle. Certainly the pace at which the disease escalated was shocking. For example on October 11, 1918, one person in Sacremento had the disease. Within a week more than two hundred cases had been reported. A week later the number was two thousand. A local paper reported that one family, the Plaices, lost three teenage sons in one night. People were ordered to wear masks in public, with violators fined between $5 and $100, or thirty days in jail.

While people searched for a cure, there was plenty of scope for weird remedies ranging from drinking castor oil to eating raw onions. It wasn't until the 1930s that anyone linked 'flu to viruses, so in 1918 no-one knew what was causing the disease, but that didn't stop wild speculation. One popular Chicago physician, Albert Croft, maintained that this was not due to an infectious organism but to "small amounts of a depressing, highly irritating, high-density gas, present in the atmosphere, especially at night".[1] Other advisors proclaimed that nakedness, fish, Germans, Chinese, open windows, closed windows or dirt were the real causes.

Hide and Seek

But as suddenly as it arrived, it disappeared. By the summer of 1920 Spanish 'flu had gone. Where? Who knows. With mass death on every side, the main priority was to bury bodies as soon as possible. Almost no-one thought to take samples of diseased tissue and attempt to preserve them for future analysis.

Recently, however, scientists have tried to focus the power of genetic analysis on three small samples. Ann Reid, Jeffery Taubenberger and colleagues at the Armed Forces Institute of Pathology, Washington, DC, chose these from lumps of tissue collected from seventy-eight servicemen who died in the 1918 pandemic. The first piece of evidence had come from a twenty-one-year-old male who came from New York State and had been stationed at Fort Jackson, South Carolina. He had become ill on September 20, 1918, and died on September 26 at 6:30 in the morning. When pathologists looked inside his chest they found clear signs of bacterial infection in his left lung, but the right lung had inflamed patches. They chopped out some of this infected tissue, soaked it in formalin to preserve it, and then embedded it in paraffin wax. The second sample came from a thirty-year-old male who had been at Camp Upton, New York. He went to the camp hospital on September 23 and died of respiratory failure, a polite phrase for suffocation, on September 26. Again pathologists cut out and preserved sections of his damaged lungs.

For the third sample Reid had to do some digging – literally. Spanish 'flu had travelled to the far north of the world, into regions where the ground is permanently frozen. Bodies buried there are effectively stored in a natural freezer and decay at incredibly slow rates. She hoped that the virus that killed so many people in Alaska would still be in the corpses.

Teller Mission (now called Brevig Mission) had suffered badly. It's a small settlement that sits on the western edge of the Seward Peninsula of Alaska, the finger tip that reaches out into the Bering Strait, and fractionally south of the polar circle. Historical records showed that in one devastating five-day period, seventy-two of the eighty-five inhabitants died. In 1997 four of these victims were exhumed from their permafrost mass grave. Although freezing a body is not the best way to preserve it if you want to study the tissue, the scientists saw clear signs of massive lung damage, bleeding and inflammation. They took samples of the tissue and returned the bodies to their icy tomb. One set of samples that came from an Inuit woman looked particularly promising.

Another 1997 expedition, which went to Longyearbyen, a Norwegian mining town on an island north of the Arctic Circle, was less successful. This team was looking for the bodies of seven fishermen and farmers who had travelled north in September 1918 hoping to make a little extra income before the ice closed in. Little did they know, but these unfortunate men had caught Spanish 'flu before leaving and they died shortly after their arrival. Their bodies still lay in graves dug in the ground and Canadian geographer Kirsty Duncan hoped that they would have been placed deep enough that the permafrost might have preserved the killer virus. Sadly, she found the likely bodies in a shallow grave, but they were too near to the thin summer sun. They had not kept well and there was no sign of the virus among the remains.

Why, you may ask, does someone want to dig around in army pathology samples and permafrost looking for such a lethal virus? The answer is unnerving. Flu pandemics have broken out at intervals throughout relatively recent history, and there is no reason why they should stop now. Before 1918 there were pandemics in 1727, 1732, 1781, 1831, 1833 and 1889. Since then there was a pandemic in 1947, Asian 'flu showed up in 1957 and Hong Kong 'flu in 1968.

Each of these outbreak years were particularly busy years for 'flu viruses, including the year of Hong Kong 'flu when more than 46,500 people were killed, sixty per cent of whom were Americans. The 1957 outbreak, which killed sixty thousand Americans, quite possibly infected more people than did the one in 1918. The death toll was lower because of antibiotics. This is not because these drugs fought off the 'flu, but because they could tackle some of the secondary infections, such as pneumonia, that took advantage of weakened people.

So at the start of the third millennium it has been quarter of a century since the last serious pandemic. All the experts agree that far from implying that such diseases are less likely, this suggests that we are due a pandemic any time now. The exact date can never be predicted, but it would be worthwhile understanding as much as we can about why particular viruses were so lethal. Then we can watch for any of these emerging within local populations and attempt to combat them.

Remarkably, Reid's work has now defined the code of five genes in the Spanish 'flu virus. Not much, you may say, if you consider that human cells possess around 20,000 genes, but this type of virus has a total of only eight. It's a lean machine. While most cells use deoxyribose nucleic acid (DNA) to store their code, these viruses use ribonucleic acid (RNA), a subtly different molecule, and they have eight small molecules of it – each molecule carries the code for a different gene.

To understand the significance of these genes we need to take a look at how 'flu viruses operate. There are basically three classes of 'flu virus, named A to C. Influenza C viruses are common, but seldom cause diseases. Influenza B viruses often cause sporadic outbreaks of disease, especially in residential communities like nursing homes. Influenza A are the nasty ones and Reid's analysis confirms that the 1918 virus was a member of this class.

Influenza A is a globe-shaped particle about a hundred nanometres in diameter. It is wrapped in a piece of cell membrane that it has ripped from the outer surface of the host cell that built it. This bilipid membrane is then studded with two different types of protein, so that the end result is something that looks like a miniature version of a war-time sea mine – and it's just about as deadly.

The two spike-like proteins are hemagglutinins and neuraminidases. The hemagglutinins help the virus get into host cells and the neuraminidases help them make good their escape. By searching through all known influenza A viruses, scientists know there are twelve different basic types of hemagglutinins, three of which (H1, H2 and H3) commonly occur in viruses that attack human cells. Similarly, there are nine neuraminidases, and N1 and N2 are in the human viruses.

When a virus approaches a cell, the hemagglutinins bind to carbo-hydrates that are protruding from the cell's surface. This isn't haphazard. The two molecules need to match much like the way that jigsaw pieces fit together. The cell then envelops the virus, holding it inside a small bubble of membrane. The fluid inside this bubble is more acid than anything the virus has encountered before and this causes the hemagglutinins to change shape. As a consequence the bubble bursts, throwing the viral RNA into the cell.

Once inside, all eight pieces of RNA set to work ordering the cell to create fresh copies of itself. New copies group together and move to the cell's membrane where the neuraminidases help wrap them in a piece of membrane. This buds off and travels away to infect another cell. In a few hours, one infected cell can generate hundreds and thousands of new viruses.

Reid's analysis shows that Spanish 'flu had hemagglutinin type 1 and neuraminidase type 1. For short hand scientists call it an H1N1 subtype. This contrasts with Asian 'flu, which is H2N2, and Hong Kong 'flu, which is H3N2. The point of interest is that while new minor variants are constantly appearing within each type of H and N, pandemics seem to occur only when a completely new H or N finds a way of getting into a virus that successfully attacks human cells.

This possibly explains why in 1976, when Private David Lewis reported sick, the world did not have a pandemic on its hands. Lewis was 18 years old and a recruit at Fort Dix, the US Army training centre in New Jersey. On January 12 he felt dizzy and nauseous. He was unusually tired, had a fever and his muscles ached. Having been there less than a week and determined to complete his training with flying colours, he ignored orders to stay in bed and joined an overnight hike, his fifty-pound pack weighing heavily on his shoulders. Needless to say, he soon lagged behind the main group and after a few hours collapsed. Lewis died shortly after arriving at the military hospital.

Lewis was just the first. By the end of January three hundred of his fellow recruits were either in hospital or confined to their beds. This caused concern. The army was well aware that Spanish 'flu had started in its ranks. New Jersey State health department director Martin Goldfield asked for samples of spit from the sufferers and an autopsy sample from Lewis. From these he established colonies of the viruses and studied them. The results were alarming. Many of the recruits had viruses bearing the dreaded H1N1 type of proteins. They had frightening similarities to Spanish 'flu.

Was this the start of a new pandemic? After all it was coming up to ten years since the last, which must mean that one was due. Soon the Centers for Disease Control and Prevention were involved. One of their virologists, Dr Walter Dowdle, confirmed that these viruses were Swine 'flu, a supposed relative of Spanish 'flu. In early February the news reached David Spencer, the CDC's director, who immediately called a meeting of top government scientists in Atlanta. They pressed the panic button and ordered that every effort should be made to develop a vaccine – and quickly.

Once you start a big machine moving it has a lot of inertia and is difficult to stop. On March 13 Spencer sent a memorandum to Capitol Hill asking for $134 million to develop and distribute a vaccine. This was despite the fact that there were indications that the epidemic was already receding. You don't ask for large sums of cash without raising interest. The words "Swine 'flu" spread faster than could any disease.

Spencer's memo caused President Ford to gather a group of experts including the inventors of the polio vaccine, Jonas Salk and Albert Sabin. The meeting was followed by a solemn television broadcast that evening. "I have been advised," said the President, "that there is a very real possibility that unless we take counteractions, there could be an epidemic of this dangerous disease next fall and winter here in the United States." He went on to announce that Congress would be asked to stump up $135 million to produce enough vaccine for every inhabitant of the United States.

Panic policies never engender good science and rarely lead to sound solutions. Immediately there were fears that a rush programme to generate a new vaccine could have disastrous consequences. After all, how would the manufacturers have time to test it? The companies asked for immunity from prosecution. Fears of a pandemic were rekindled in late July when almost two hundred members of the American Legion fell ill at a convention in Philadelphia. The CDC quickly showed that this "Legionnaire's Disease" was different from the Swine 'flu virus. It took more than a year to track the cause of this outbreak to bacteria in the air-conditioning system. The shock of more deaths, and among such a prestigious group of people, was sufficient to grant the companies their desired immunity. It was set out in a piece of ill-conceived legislation that was rushed through congress in August that year.

Two hundred million doses were needed, but an element of chaos started creeping into the pharmaceutical industry. One company, Parke-Davis, even succeeded in making two million doses of vaccine targeted at the wrong strain of virus.[2]

The vaccination campaign started in earnest on October 1, despite reports that the vaccine had only limited usefulness. But when two elderly people died shortly after receiving their jabs the press went wild. President Ford passionately pleaded for the American people to ignore the scare and step forward and his publicists worked hard to fill the papers with photos of Ford and his wife receiving the jab. Only about a quarter of the population took heed and followed the call.

The final nail in the coffin of the vaccination effort came when people started claiming that the vaccine triggered Guillian-Barré syndrome, a nervous disease that sometimes follows viral illnesses. The first case appeared in Minnesota in the third week of November and was quickly followed by others. By Christmas Day the CDC had 172 cases on their books, ninety-nine of which seemed to be linked to the vaccine. Six had died. By New Year the number of vaccine-related cases had risen to 257. Doctors also recorded a further 269 cases in which they could find no direct link with the vaccine. The list of vaccine-related victims eventually reached more than eleven hundred, with all states being represented. Fifty-eight people had died.

Guillian-Barré syndrome was not new and a normal rate of disease would have seen some two hundred people affected by the disease in any one year. The lawyers loved it and soon 4,181 claims were filed, seeking a total of $3.2 billion. It's reasonable to assume that the pharmaceutical companies were relieved they had pressed for immunity and the US government handed out the best part of $100 million in compensation over the following couple of decades.

As the dust settled on 1976 it became known as a year of remarkable good health. Not because of the vaccination effort, but because of the remarkably low level of viruses circulating in the population. The epidemic had not materialised. The whole exercise had been a waste of time – except that it showed policy makers plenty of ways that they could improve on things in the future.

With more knowledge of viral infection, it now appears that the epidemic was never going to happen precisely because the H1N1 type of virus had been seen before. To establish mass disease you need a virus where either the H or the N type has never been seen before. If either is new, the body's defence system doesn't recognise the virus in time and it can thrive. An old virus will be spotted, and dealt with, in at least enough people to prevent epidemic levels of disease.

But we can't relax. A leopard might not be able to change its spots, but viruses have proved that they are very capable of changing their spikes. There is no reason why a new version shouldn't appear. In fact, there is every reason to suspect that it could.

Origins – Past and Future

New pandemics might appear to have no previous history, but the virus hasn't appeared from thin air. It is not a brand new act of creation on the part of a malicious deity. A key problem for the virus detectives chasing the 1918 agent is to work out where it came from. The issue boils down to three options: was its origin human, avian (from birds) or porcine (from pigs)? Their concern is not just with the origins of past epidemics, but that we have an idea of where future disease may originate.

Host cells that give residence to viruses are great melting pots for RNA viruses. Each gene comes on its own snippet of RNA, so if a cell becomes infected by more than one type of virus there is every opportunity for a molecular game of mix and match. Pigs seem to be a good intermediate for many viruses. In terms of their biology, they are remarkably similar to human beings, but also similar to other non-human animals. As a result they have the potential to act like a bridge.

To perform this function, the pigs need to live in close proximity to both humans and birds. China provides just such an environment. Viruses are masterful quick-change artists, and Chinese farming practices provide an ideal place for them. Chickens are farmed alongside fish farms where ducks swim on the ponds, and pig manure is often thrown in as fish food. The farmer lives in the middle of all this activity. Viruses can take their pick from the genetic soup, borrowing from the pool of pathogens that prior to these farming methods have been much more restricted to a single breed of animal.

This may well have happened in May 1997 when a three-year-old boy in Hong Kong died of influenza. When the CDC investigated this death they found that the causal virus was unique. It was Influenza A – no surprise there – but subtype H5N1. Never before had H5 been part of a human-infecting virus. The alarm bells sounded.

Hong Kong imports around seventy-five thousand chickens a day from mainland China. It turned out that this virus had been killing chickens in the area for some time, but no-one had worried about human health because they knew the virus and the acquired wisdom was that H5 didn't touch us. They were wrong.

In a radical step to stamp out the disease, Hong Kong's authorities ordered the slaughter of 1.4 million birds and banned any imports of live chickens. The import ban was only lifted in January 1998 amid controversy as to whether the virus originated in China or in the unsanitary conditions of many of Hong Kong's poultry facilities. Fortunately this virus didn't cause a mass disease, though it did raise considerable concern and seventeen other cases were eventually reported, six of which ended in the person's death.

March 1999 brought more bad news for Chinese/Hong Kong chickens. Influenza A subtype H9N2 made itself at home in two Hong Kong children. Once again a type of hemagglutinin only reported in birds had made its way into a human virus. One victim was a one-year-old and the other a four-year-old. They had classic signs of viral 'flu, with difficulty breathing and high fevers. Both recovered, but the world's health authorities had some more sleepless nights. By April there were no more reports of infections with this mutant agent, but Hong Kong and international health agencies kept a close eye on the situation.

A meeting in the UK on April 13, 1999, concluded that there was little to be worried about with H9N2 and that there was no evidence that this variant of 'flu was about to trigger a pandemic. These same reassuring scientists, however, also set in motion plans to build a vaccine against the virus – as a precautionary measure – just in case. But this wasn't the end of bird 'flu.

Researchers looking into the 1918 pandemic had already made the link between the disease and pig farming. All of the army recruits who triggered fresh outbreaks when they arrived at their training bases had come from pig farms. More recently immunological detective work has added weight to this argument.

When a virus invades a person's body it moves inside host cells. The

RNA replicates and starts to make proteins that the cell has never seen before. Machinery inside the cell grabs samples of all proteins produced, chops it up and then presents it on the outside of the cell so that white blood cells can take a look at it. They are programmed to get aggressive if they encounter proteins that they have never seen before and on seeing a viral protein are liable to attack and destroy the infected cell. These white cells also respond in a similarly destructive way if they find a virus floating around. Once they've seen a particular type of foreign particle they cause the body to build many more white cells tuned to the task of hunting out these critters.

The problem is that it takes time for the body to build an army of defenders and in a fast moving illness like the 1918 disease you could easily be dead before you've built a big enough force. If you survive, however, your blood will always carry cells alerted to that particular virus, ready and waiting for action. It's the basis of vaccination – show the immune system a little of a weakened form of the disease and it will be ready to protect you against infection should the real thing come along.

The first time a baby faces a 'flu virus the response is large and it leaves an indelible mark on his or her immune system. Scientists call it original viral sin. Searching through blood samples from people born between 1918 and 1920 shows that for many the original sinner was a virus that looked remarkably like Swine Influenza A H1N1. More evidence that Spanish 'flu came from pigs. The question then is, how had the pig encountered this virus? Well, Influenza A is rife among ducks in Canada that migrate south. Quite possibly a 'flu-infected duck had dropped faeces in a Kansas farm. Pigs had picked it up and passed it to humans.

The story looked simple until Reid and Taubenberger added their RNA code data from the 1918 tissue samples into the equation. By comparing the genetic code taken from the victims with that of other known viruses you can build up a picture of the viral family tree. Each generation of virus should show small changes from the ones immediately before and after it, so after a lot of detective work it is possible to place viruses in some form of chronological order. Also the rate of change is fairly constant, so by comparing swine-infecting viruses with those in humans, you can get an impression of how long it has been since they moved species.

Weighing all the information indicates that the virus had probably entered humans between 1900 and 1915, some years before the epidemic. When viruses enter a new host species their genetic code undergoes rapid changes, and while the H and N proteins remain of the same type, they

1-Smallpox could go down in history as the first disease to be deliberately eradicated − "could" because stocks of the virus are deliberately held in labs in the US and Russia. Let's hope they never escape, because with vaccination wound down, no one in the world is immune. This electron micrograph has been coloured to show the protein coat in yellow and the virus's DNA in red (x28500 magnification).

2-On 26 October 1977, Somalian cook Ali Maow Maalin found fame when he became the last known person to catch smallpox from viruses in the wild. He is also unusual in that he survived to tell the tale.

3-The Ebola virus strikes fear in anyone who knows its power to kill. This re-worked transmission electron micrograph shows its characteristic string-like shape.

4-By finding that many diseases are caused by infectious micro agents, Louis Pasteur revolutionised medicine.

5-Mention the discovery of antibiotics and Alexander Fleming's name is more likely to spring to mind than any other. Here he is holding his famous penicillin culture plate. While he was the first to observe this wonder chemical in action, he was unable to capture its power and turn the compound into a germ-fighting drug.

6-Ernest Chain (above) and Howard Florey (overleaf) are the two names that you should remember in association with antibiotic discovery. Their knowledge of chemistry and sheer determination made penicillin a household name at the end of the Second World War.

7-Howard Florey.

8-Anton van Leewenhoek created some of the earliest microscopes and was the first person to describe micro-organisms such as protozoa and bacteria. Little did he know that some of his "little living animalcules" would turn out to be killers.

9-The eyes and antennae of a female *anopheles gambia* mosquito –
in itself a fairly innocuous beast, but a member of the disease hall of
fame by virtue of the insect's ability to transmit malaria.

10-The plague terrorised fourteenth-century Europe, massacring
millions of men, women and children, rich and poor, as
Jan Brueghel the younger depicted in his masterpiece entitled
the "Triumph of Death". The painting draws extensively from
one created by his father Pieter Brueghel the elder, which
currently hangs in the Museo del Prado, Madrid.
That generation may be long-since dead, but the disease
lives on. 1998 saw a strain of plague bacteria emerge in
Madagascar that was resistant to almost all known antibiotics.

11-Saint Roch prays to Mary in Jacques Louis David's painting. The hermit's petition is that Mary should intervene and end the plague.

12-Polio destroys nerves and thus paralyses muscles. If it affects the chest the victim can't breathe. An Iron lungs provides a negative pressure around the patient's chest and helps the person survive.

Thanks to PENICILLIN
...He Will Come Home!

★ ★

FROM ORDINARY MOLD—
the Greatest Healing Agent of this War!

© 1944

On the gaudy, green-and-yellow mold above, called *Penicillium notatum* in the laboratory, grows the miraculous substance first discovered by Professor Alexander Fleming in 1928. Named penicillin by its discoverer, it is the most potent weapon ever developed against many of the deadliest infections known to man. Because research on molds was already a part of Schenley enterprise, Schenley Laboratories were well able to meet the problem of large-scale production of penicillin, when the great need for it arose.

When the thunderous battles of this war have subsided to pages of silent print in a history book, the greatest news event of World War II may well be the discovery and development — *not* of some vicious secret weapon that *destroys* — but of a weapon that *saves* lives. That weapon, of course, is penicillin.

Every day, penicillin is performing some unbelievable act of healing on some far battlefront. Thousands of men will return home who otherwise would not have had a chance. Better still, more and more of this precious drug is now available for civilian use... to save the lives of patients of every age.

A year ago, production of penicillin was difficult, costly. Today, due to specially-devised methods of mass-production, in use by Schenley Laboratories, Inc. and the 20 other firms designated by the government to make penicillin, it is available in ever-increasing quantity, at progressively lower cost.

Listen to "THE DOCTOR FIGHTS" starring RAYMOND MASSEY. Tuesday evenings, C.B.S. See your paper for time and station.

SCHENLEY LABORATORIES, INC.
Lawrenceburg, Indiana
Producers of PENICILLIN-*Schenley*

★ ★

13-The rapid build-up of resistance to penicillin was accelerated all the more because it was available without prescription. This advert from the August 14,1944, edition of *Life* magazine carried the unspoken message that penicillin is an inexpensive wonder drug – take it often.

14-Looking like a lunar landing module, bacteriophage T4 locks on to the outside of a bacterial cell – in this case a blue-stained *E.coli*. Its legs squat down, causing a tube to pierce the bacterial wall and allowing the virus's DNA to gain entry. Once on board, the DNA turns the unwitting bacterium into a virus-producing factory.

15-ABOVE: The 1919 'flu epidemic killed twice as many people as died in World War One. By wearing masks some people hoped to evade its evil spell.

16-Anthrax and bubonic plague stand a high possibility of being used as a terrorist weapon. Right-wing American activist Larry Wayne Harris also showed that it was relatively easy to get hold of both of these organisms and only a lack of patience on his part led to his arrest and incarceration.

17- We live in a global village, one in which distance no longer acts as a barrier to the spread of disease. If in doubt visit New York. July 28, 2000 was just another day in that summer, a summer when tons of insecticide were pumped into the air to kill mosquitoes, because the mosquitoes were transmitting West Nile Virus. The virus had probably "emigrated" from Israel.

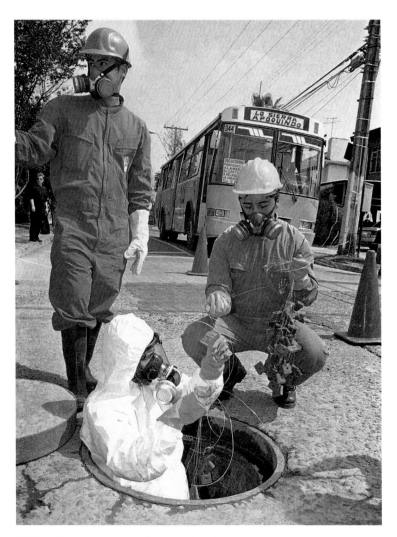

18-Hanta Virus causes symptoms that are similar to flu, but the death-rate is higher. It is spread by fleas on rodents, so when an outbreak hit Santiago, Chile in September 1994 there was a rush to clear the vermin from their sewers.

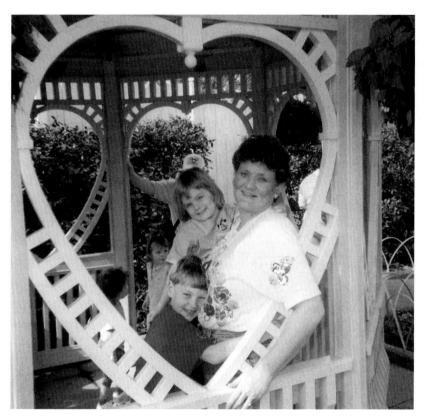

19-Rita is remarkable. She is one of the few people to survive a full-blown attack of *Streptococcus B,* an attack that tore massive chunks out of her legs and put her in a coma for 18 days. Her young children feared that they would never see their mother again.

20- In 1994 the author met a team of professional sex
workers in Cheredzi, a sugar-producing town in the
south east of Zimbabwe. These women had been trained
to perform songs and dramas that give stark messages:
Sexual intercourse transmits HIV, the virus that causes
AIDS. AIDS kills. The safest sex is abstinence, but failing
that, use a condom. Their message is all the more
poignant as most of them would be carrying the virus.

become subtly altered. The theory now is that the virus moved from an aquatic bird to pigs and from there to humans. Once on board a human being, it mutated from a version that was not particularly virulent or infectious to one that could spread easily. This level of mutation coincided with the mass call to arms and gave the virus access to millions of new people. Out in the wide world, the virus had a fresh opportunity to mutate and by the autumn had turned into a killer. The rest is history.

The interest, however, doesn't stop there. If this killer bug came from ancestral viruses in waterfowl or pigs, then it or its close relative could easily still be out there. The 1918 'flu pandemic may have come to an abrupt end, but until we understand the exact make up of the virus we will never be able to understand why it had such a dramatic effect. Until we know where it came from, we will never be sure where to look to spot a new version breaking out.

You can also see the reason for the concern about the new Hong Kong viruses. It may well be that they are not particularly virulent. For the moment we are safe. But if they have established themselves in human beings, albeit at a very low level, they will have the opportunity of slowly mutating. It happened in 1918.

Escalating Alert

From 2001 to 2004, the western world's attention in terms of defending itself from terrifying threats became focused on terror networks. Western lives and lifestyles seemed to be under threat and the response was hard and fast. First Afghanistan and then Iraq felt the force of the assault, aimed at tearing the heart out of what President George W. Bush famously called the "axis of evil". This may have been a fatal distraction, because in the background the 'flu viruses in the East were learning new tricks.

A 2005 editorial in the scientific journal *Nature* began with an apocalyptic warning: "Millions of people killed in highly developed countries within months. Tens of millions worldwide. The global economy in tatters. A Hollywood fantasy? No – it's now a plausible scenario. The first act… has already started across Asia. Unless the international community now moves decisively to mitigate this pandemic threat, we will in all probability pay heavily within a few years. Then, hard questions will be asked as to why we were not prepared."[3]

The fear again stems from 'flu. In February 2003, a novel strain of bird 'flu broke out in the Netherlands. This version was H7N7 and the Dutch authorities acted swiftly. By April they had culled eleven million birds –

about ten per cent of the country's poultry flock. The virus seemed mainly confined to birds, but not exclusively so. More than 80 people contracted mild eye infections caused by the virus and some had additional 'flu-like symptoms. These were mainly people involved in the cull, but, worryingly, two of those affected caught the virus from infected family members. One of these was a twelve-year-old child. The clear message was that the virus had the potential of travelling between humans. More worrying still was the death of a fifty-seven-year-old veterinarian who had been working with the infected flocks. The outbreak served as a warning that avian 'flu viruses are quite capable of mutating and gaining hold even in highly developed and regulated agricultural systems.

While Europe was getting its first taste of the disease, the East was experiencing yet more varieties breaking into the human population. A child with 'flu in Hong Kong was found to have the H9N2 variant of the virus. Now this raises another question. Is the occasional human infection with a weird virus a new phenomenon, or something that increased vigilance means that we are only now detecting? The answer is probably the latter – this has probably been going on for as long as viruses have existed. But that is no grounds for relaxing. The chance of any one virus breaching a species barrier and jumping, for example from duck to human, is slim. But viruses have had millions of years to try it, and occasionally they succeed. While few of these viruses have the additional capability of spreading ferociously, it potentially only needs one to make the jump to have a crisis.

With much of the world's media still obsessed with the crisis in Iraq, few agencies gave much coverage to the January 2004 announcement that lab tests had confirmed that H5N1 had taken hold in Vietnam. The infection was rife in the poultry flock, had killed over 40,000 birds, and had already infected fourteen people, killing twelve of them. Health officials were relieved that there was no sign of the virus being transmitted from person to person.

In the last week of January 2004, the Indonesian authorities stopped denying that their flocks had the virus and admitted that it had been spreading since the previous August.[4] Thailand stepped up and also admitted that the government there had known that the virus was in Thai flocks since November. Chinese officials claimed that they had only spotted the infection that week, although in reality the virus may have originated in China early in 2003. These sorts of denials come because of the economic impact. Not only does recognition of the disease lead to pressures for a massive and costly cull, it also means that the country loses huge international orders for frozen meals containing chicken. Not many people realise when they take a frozen meal from a supermarket counter how far this bird meat may have flown.

An editorial in the weekly science magazine *New Scientist* summed up the situation: "The bird 'flu sweeping Asia has achieved near-uncontrollable dimensions, and the reason is clear: several countries have been covering up infections for months. Did we learn nothing from SARS about the folly of concealing disease? Well, health ministries might have. But bird 'flu affects poultry, at least to start with, and agriculture ministries protect farming and trade, and think short-term. They are less likely to admit a problem until forced to."[5]

Vietnam then announced another nasty twist in the tale. In February 2004, they had evidence that two women had caught bird 'flu from other people. Investigations showed that a thirty-one-year-old man and his sister had prepared duck for the meal at a wedding celebration. Both of them became infected with the bird 'flu virus and the sister died shortly after the event. The man's wife and another of his sisters came to the wedding and both caught the virus – the wife died. There is no evidence that either of these women had had direct contact with poultry, so they must have contracted bird 'flu second-hand from the infected humans.

And on it goes. In January 2005, there was the announcement that two more people in Vietnam had contracted H5N1 bird 'flu virus, bringing the death total in that country to seven and leaving at least seven others infected. Small numbers, yes, but the devil is all too often in the detail. The critical issue here was that two of the people now in hospital had caught the virus not from an animal, but from another infected human.

The implications of human-to-human transmission are severe. You may be able to contain an animal-borne disease by wiping out all of the livestock, but no society would contemplate massacring large proportions of its population on the basis that the individuals might be infected with a virus. If the virus has really picked up, or generated, genes that enable it to move from human to human, then we are moving into a worrying phase of this outbreak.

One other natural event that made the 'flu epidemic more dangerous was the tsunami that struck the islands and shorelines of the Indian Ocean on Boxing Day 2004. While the tidal wave killed well over 150,000 people, it had another, possibly more dangerous, effect. The tsunami not only captured the attention of the press, it also monopolised the attention of the public health systems in the affected countries. A consequence of this is that the exercise of vigilance on avian 'flu all but stopped. This shift of attention could prove costly in the long term.

Writing in the *British Medical Journal*, one doctor highlights the issue: "The tsunami in Asia illustrated one acute natural trauma with thousands of deaths. That catastrophe pales into insignificance when compared with an influenza pandemic. Hundreds of millions will die if the world does not act to prevent this developing pandemic."[6]

A strange waiting game developed through 2005. Virus hunters at the heart of the action kept sending out alerts about new sightings as this virus roamed South East Asia, but on a global scale few people paid any attention. Then in October, H5N1 bird flu reached Europe and killed more than 1,000 birds on a farm in Turkey. Officials quickly culled other birds near that village. Then a Romanian village in the Danube delta, which is a stopover for migratory birds from Asia, was quarantined after 36 birds died. They too had 'flu. But still the real threat hadn't materialised. Yes, birds were infecting birds and many were dying. A few humans were catching the disease, but the virus wasn't passing from person to person – at least not yet.

At last policy makers started to take notice. Delegates from eighty nations and international agencies met in Washington DC to see what could be done about bird 'flu. "The world is clearly unprepared, or inadequately prepared, for a pandemic of H5N1 influenza," said US Health and Human Services Secretary Mike Leavitt. But realising the depth of the problem can be a good starting point for action.

Throwing Up Defences

The surprising, maybe even frightening, thing is that with all our advances in medicine we are only a little more prepared to fight off a new 'flu pandemic now than we were in 1918. Antibiotics might help combat secondary bacterial infections, but they don't touch viruses, which we have few means of attacking. Any chemical that tries to stop viral reproduction would have to act on, and probably kill, the host cells. Those host cells are the very ones that make up our bodies. Generally not a good idea to kill them. In limited situations this can work: it is, for example, the way that external chemical treatments are used to get rid of warts and verrucas. You apply some noxious chemical, kill the skin cells and the virus that triggers the growth has nowhere to live. It drops off with the dead tissue. This, however, would not be a good approach to treating a wide-ranging lung infection. So, to find an antiviral agent, you need to identify processes that are unique to viral replication – this is not easy, but a few contenders are just coming to the market.

Vaccination

One defensive shield that we have now is vaccination – the ability to make a solution containing either weakened versions of the disease agent, or fragments of the agent's protein shell. Every autumn in western countries, doctors offer 'flu vaccines to elderly people and others at risk of serious complications should they get a bout of 'flu. The UK health authorities recommend that anyone over sixty-five has an annual dose, as well as those with diabetes, heart disease, chronic kidney disease or asthma.

A few problems make this vaccination against 'flu a less than ideal solution. The first is that in any one year there are tens of 'flu viruses circulating around the world in low numbers. In the current global market place 'flu planners can't ignore a virus just because it happens to be on the other side of the world. One plane trip could alter that. Unfortunately, it isn't possible to build a vaccine targeted at more than a few different viruses, so the decision-makers must scratch their heads each summer and try to predict which versions are likely to dominate in the following winter. It's guided guesswork, and there is no guarantee that they will get it right. A rank outsider could always creep up on the blind-side and win the pandemic stakes.

Then there is the problem of out-and-out newcomers. Surveillance systems around the world are improving, but you can't detect anything until someone not only gets infected but also becomes ill. There are a huge number of viruses in circulation that do little or no harm, and it's not an easy job spotting the ones that might suddenly turn nasty. Since there is no way you could build and store a vaccine targeted at them all, you've just got to rely again on best guesses.

Speaking on the US Public Broadcasting Service in December 1997, David Heymann, Director of the Programme on Emerging and other Communicable Diseases for the WHO indicated another problem. He was answering questions on the current Hong Kong chicken 'flu and was asked how the development of a 'flu vaccine was going. His answer was revealing: "Well, this virus is a very lethal virus, and, therefore it can't be grown on eggs, which normally viruses grow on to produce vaccines." Remember, viruses can only grow in number if they can infect living cells. Hen eggs are great little incubators for viruses in that they are sterile inside, have a lump of fast growing cells (the embryo) and a lot of nutrients. If, however, the virus kills the embryo too quickly, then there is no time for its numbers to increase.

Heymann explained that scientists were working to develop a virus that, as far as the human immune system was concerned, would look identical to the chicken 'flu virus, but that would also grow on eggs. This can take months to achieve, again highlighting the need to be forewarned about a possible pandemic. If a disease moves fast, you may not have months to gear up and develop stocks. The average time from the start of work to the arrival of a 'flu vaccine is currently six months, a lag period that industry is working hard at reducing.

Vaccines are also not as good as the real thing. They give some protection, and for people who are in high-risk groups, the 'flu jab is a good idea. All the same, getting the disease gives greater protection than the vaccine, but the problem is that the disease may kill.

This then raises the thorny issue of the safety of vaccines. The 1976 experience in the USA, where vaccination induced Guillian-Barré syndrome, did little to inspire confidence. Many lessons have been learned and modern vaccines are much safer. Having a jab is a social as well as a personal decision, because vaccination campaigns work best when there is good uptake. It's not easy to calculate the exact percentage of people who need to be vaccinated to prevent a disease moving within populations, but the idea is to have a sufficiently high number of resistant people within the community that any virus that enters is effectively isolated. With nowhere to go, the disease dies out. At best, it is never seen again. At worst, it returns to the non-human animal reservoir from whence it came, ready for another attempt should the appropriate chain of events come about in the future.

That said, as the bird 'flu epidemic gained pace in the East, many countries started to vaccinate the birds in their poultry flock. At first sight this makes economic as well as ethical sense. The question that only history will answer is whether it makes scientific sense. The problem is that no vaccine is 100 per cent effective, and what could easily happen is that it keeps the level of virus down to a level that is deemed acceptable, without eradicating it. This is just what a would-be viral terror-chief would love. With the virus lurking in the background, it has all the time it likes to evolve.

Mass vaccination of humans runs a similar, though this time greater, risk. You could easily generate a situation where the virus moves into the human population and spreads around without causing any mass outbreaks of disease. By living inside human cells, however, the virus is very likely to bump into others that have learned more savage tricks, such as HIV or other 'flu viruses. These chance encounters give the virus the possibility of acquiring new bits of DNA, new chunks of genetic instructions that can enable it to take an evolutionary leap. Vaccination is certainly not going to be a quick fix.

Antivirals

If vaccination doesn't work, then there is a slowly growing range of pharmaceutical agents on the market that offer some help. None of them have the power of antibiotics to kill the infective agent, but they do look increasingly hopeful.

There is no point in trying to block the cell's metabolism and thereby impede the virus's reproductive cycle because nothing in that part of the particle's "life-cycle" is unique. Any drug that blocked protein synthesis, for example, would kill the host. But there are two unique steps – entry and exit.

Influenza A viruses can do nothing on their own. The only way a virus manages to get into its target cells is by brushing up against it, and allowing the cell to grab it, wrap it in a section of membrane and drag this vesicle inside. The cell's aim is to clear the virus out of circulation and then to destroy it, but once inside the cell, the virus does the only thing it can – it releases the genetic material stored in the virus, and then lets this material take command of just enough of the cell's internal machinery so that the cell generates many more viruses. Amantadine, and its derivative rimantadine, work by making it harder for the virus to shed its genetic material from the vesicle. The virus effectively becomes trapped in the cell and locked safely away. It's only effective on Influenza A viruses and then only when given before the person gets infected.

One Canadian study showed how the drug could be used in a residential home for elderly people. [7] As soon as one resident became ill with 'flu, the rest were given amantadine and this proved to be seventy to ninety per cent effective. It's not an easy process, though, because amantadine's other use is to help people with Parkinson's Disease, and as such it can have neurological side effects such as dizziness, nausea, hallucinations and character change. To minimise the chance of this occurring, medical staff need to work out for each patient how well their kidneys are working, and then use this information to adjust the dose. This demands considerable preparation and careful drug delivery.

According to this study, the other problem is that amantadine-resistant viruses can emerge even during a short course of treatment, which can lead to new cases of influenza.

The other approach is to allow viruses into cells, but to block their exit. This is the approach taken by zanamivir, a drug marketed by GlaxoSmithKline as Relenza, and Roche's drug oseltamivir, which they market under the trade name Tamiflu. The drug goes straight to the lung lining, the place where the viruses are most active, and blocks neuraminidase, the protein in the virus's coat that enables it to break out of the cells. This means that the first viruses get into your body and start to reproduce inside your cells, but if it is caught early enough you can stop the infection getting worse. This also means that the chance of the infection being passed on to others is reduced. The downside is that the treatment must be taken within 48 hours of the initial infection, which means you have to act quickly. Such haste reduces the physician's chance of saying, "Go to bed for a couple of days and come back if you are still unwell" – as by then it will be too late to start the drug. The manufacturers claim that drugs like these shorten the duration of symptoms. Some trials show that this reduction is in the order of one day. In 2000, a course of treatment cost somewhere around $75.

The silver lining in the so-called "war on terror" may be an increased preparedness to fight a 'flu pandemic. The fear that some disaffected terror organisation could deliberately unleash a virus in a major city has led to fresh pressure for stockpiles of drugs. In 2004, the UK government ordered 14.6 million doses of anti-viral drugs. The idea was that this stockpile should be built up over the following two years. US health planners believe they have stockpiles capable of treating more than forty million people. It's a step in the right direction, but it is hardly a policy decision that will prevent a pandemic.

At a WHO conference in Geneva in December 2004, experts tried to put a number on the expected loss of life if 'flu broke out as a pandemic. Unsurprisingly, putting a group of experts in a room was unlikely to yield a clear-cut conclusion, and their estimates varied from two million to fifty million dead, with many times that number needing medical assistance. The estimates might cover a broad range – but none of them were pleasant to contemplate. One thing they did agree on was that you can't stop the spread of a pandemic, but if you are prepared for it you can reduce its impact.

Confusing mild winter bugs with 'flu gives us a false sense of security. Real 'flu is a killer and the bottom line is that 'flu viruses are smart. They stay predominantly in single animal populations, but occasionally break out and cause havoc in new hosts. We are reasonably good at tracking them, getting better at developing vaccines, but have a long way to go before we have a powerful cure.

CHAPTER 7 - SARS - OVERDUE PANDEMIC OR ALARMIST PANIC?

The first that almost anyone had heard of SARS was a short news item in the February 14, 2003 edition of *The Weekly Epidemiological Record*, the global germ-watchers' newsletter. It read: "Health officials from Guangdong Province have reported a total of 305 cases and five deaths of acute respiratory syndrome between 16 November and 9 February 2003. A team from the Chinese Ministry of Health is working with Guangdong health officials to investigate the outbreak and collect samples for laboratory analysis."[1] The article continued by saying that there was no evidence that 'flu viruses were involved, and that they felt the worst was over. This assessment got one point right and one wrong: it wasn't 'flu, but it was far from over. Two weeks later, another article in the same newsletter, suggested that the mystery killer was probably the yeast organism, *Chlamydia pneumoniae*.[2] Wrong again.

The story of severe acute respiratory syndrome, nicknamed SARS by someone who then became a victim of its killing power, started on November 16, 2002 when a father of four went into hospital in Foshan, China, a heavily populated area where factories intermingle with shrimp, pig and duck farms.[3] He had a respiratory illness that was in many ways like pneumonia. The illness seemed unremarkable and the man recovered and went home. End of story – one well man. Not quite.

The identity of this man has been kept a closely guarded secret, because while he has survived, hundreds of people who met the virus he was harbouring were much less fortunate. "You wouldn't want your medical records released, would you?" said WHO team spokesman Chris Powell when reporters wanted to know more.[4] All reporters could discover was that the man was in his forties and lived in Foshan. What else is clear is that, while he may have been relatively unaffected by the disease, others in the area were soon seriously ill and some were dying.

While the disease was contained in China, few people in the rest of the world either knew or cared about it. But then it went walkabout.

On February 21, 2003, Liu Jianlun checked into room 911 on the ninth floor of the Metropole Hotel in Hong Kong's Kowloon district. He was sixty-four, and was the professor of nephrology at Zhongshan University, but over the past few weeks had spent much of his time treating people with a mystery bug.[5] Liu had travelled to Hong Kong to attend a wedding, and had felt slightly unwell for a few days before his trip. Waking on the next day, he felt seriously ill and, too sick to attend the wedding, took himself off to the local Kwong Wah Hospital.

In doing this he triggered a chain of events that would be repeated across the globe, in which healthcare workers and patients found themselves in severe danger of contracting the disease and passing it on to family and friends. As such, hospitals swapped over from being centres of health to dispensaries of disease.

With a month or so's experience of the disease, Liu recognised his symptoms and immediately told hospital staff that he was highly infectious and needed to wear a mask to prevent passing the disease on. Members of the hospital staff were less convinced. But he went further, asking to be placed in an isolation unit behind double-sealed doors with reduced air pressure. By the time he died on March 4, the doctors and nurses were taking his pleas more seriously.

If Liu had taken the virus only to the local hospital, life in the rest of the world would quite possibly have been left undisturbed. But he had stayed one night in the hotel, and seven other visitors to the ninth floor of the hotel soon became victims, along with his brother-in-law and two nurses at the hospital.

The first known casualty was 48-year-old American businessman, Johnny Chen. He had stayed at the Metropole before flying out to Hanoi, Vietnam, on February 24. It was a business trip: he worked for an import-export company. Five days after sharing an elevator with Liu, Chen became ill, and on February 26 went to the Vietnam-France Hospital in Hanoi. Clearly he was very sick. Two days later, Chen was visited by fifty-three-year-old Carlo Urbani, an infectious disease expert who had been called to Hanoi from the World Health Organisation's Asian office in Bangkok. He soon realised that Chen had a hitherto unknown condition and named it SARS.[6] No one knew what it was, but giving it a name made it seem more real. Within days Urbani realised that Chen was not alone, and alerted the WHO to unusual numbers of atypical pneumonia in the Vietnam-France Hospital.

Having been ill for eleven days, Chen was air-evacuated back to Hong Kong and taken straight to the Princess Margaret Hospital, a move which enabled the virus to make itself at home in a second Hong Kong hospital. While Chen might have left Hanoi, the bug stayed on. By March 8, fourteen staff at the Vietnam-France Hospital were ill. Help was needed, and a WHO team arrived to bring expert assistance. Two days later and new cases were showing every day – 22 of the staff were now sick and the tally was rising.

On March 11, Urbani left for Bangkok where he was due to give a presentation on tropical diseases. Ironically, having given this disease the name SARS, it now came back and bit him. Almost as soon as he arrived, he found himself in another hospital, this time as the patient – he had caught the disease while trying to save the lives of others. The next day the WHO put out a world alert drawing everyone's attention to this disease.[7]

Two days later Chen died in his Hong Kong hospital bed, but not before the bug had jumped from him to many other people along his travels, originating new outbreaks. Urbani died on March 29, one month and a day after he had first met Chen. WHO representative in Vietnam Pascale Brudon praised his late colleague, saying, "When people became very concerned in the hospital, he was there every day, collecting samples, talking to the staff and strengthening infection control procedures." Urbani was not blind to the risk that his work involved. He had explained the situation to Giuliana his wife: "If I can't work in such situations, what am I here for? Answering e-mails, going to cocktail parties and pushing paper?" But the tragedy doesn't end with his death as his wife and three children, Tommaso, Luca and Maddalena live to mourn his loss.

Another early victim was a twenty-six-year-old Hong Kong airport worker who visited an acquaintance on the Metropole Hotel's dreaded ninth floor. He fell sick on February 24 and was treated in ward 8A of the Prince of Wales Hospital.[8] Now the virus had checked in at its third hospital in Hong Kong, infecting staff who in turn went home and infected their families. In retrospect, it is unfortunate that the doctors treated him using a jet nebuliser. And they were thorough; he had it four times a day for seven days. You can see why they did it, as spraying moisture into someone's lungs is often a very good way of helping them breathe if their lungs are infected. In this case, however, it served to generate a cloud of infectious droplets that wafted around the hospital ward. Breathe it in, or let it land on the watery covering of your eye, and you invite the virus into your body.

The SARS virus soon showed that it held no respect for rank, as William Ho, chief executive of the Hong Kong hospital authority, was admitted to hospital on Sunday, March 23 and by the following Tuesday was confirmed to have the disease.[9]

Hitch-hiking Around the Globe

Infectious diseases do not need passports to move around, but they do need people and Kwan Sui-chu provided the SARS-causing agent free passage to Canada. "The SARS virus travels at the speed of a jumbo jet," commented Shigeru Omi, the WHO's regional director for the Western Pacific.[10] Toronto residents, Kwan and her husband had travelled to Hong Kong to visit their son and had stayed in the Metropole in order to make use of the free five-night voucher that came with their airline ticket. It turned out to be a costly freebie – their room was on the ninth floor.

With the trip over, Kwan flew home to Toronto on February 23, and by February 26 was feeling decidedly ill. She died at home and was buried without an autopsy. And why not? Kwan was seventy-eight and had diabetes; who needed any more information as to why she had died of a 'flu-like illness? That was until on March 5, Kwan's forty-four-year-old son, Tse Chi Kwai, his wife and their baby went to their family doctor all complaining of a respiratory disease. Next day, Tse went to the Scarborough Grace Hospital – the institution that subsequently became the centre of Canada's outbreak.

Doctors initially thought he had pneumonia – a diagnosis that made sense of most of his symptoms. While he waited to be admitted to a hospital ward, he lay next to a seventy-six-year-old man with an unsteady heartbeat. Three days later, Tse was getting no better and the doctors moved him to an isolation ward. By now they suspected that he might have tuberculosis. For the first time hospital staff started using protection. After all, no one wants to catch TB. His family wore masks when they came to see him and washed their hands as they left, but by now the genie was out of the bottle. Tse died on March 12. Four days later the man with the dicky heart was back in hospital with breathing problems. He died on March 22 and the World Health Organisation raised the alert.[11] A further eleven people in Canada were suspected of having the illness. Toronto was in the news.

Within days, some of the medical staff who had had contact with Tse and family started feeling ill and so did members of their families. The virus had moved into Toronto and the world was holding its breath.

At the same time people were beginning to think again about travelling to places that seemed to be SARS hotbeds. The American Association for

Cancer Research had spent a year planning its annual meeting due to run from April 5 to 9, with the venue as Toronto. As March turned into April, the Association found itself receiving a steady stream of cancellations. Attending an academic medical conference may be fun, it may even be informative, but it was not something to risk your life over. And people were beginning to question the safety of travelling to what was becoming seen as a world centre of disease.

The AACR had received 6,900 abstracts, booked 400 speakers, and expected about 16,000 participants, but faced with the prospect of having too many empty stages and meeting-rooms, the association pulled the plug on April 2. "Cancelling the meeting was a difficult decision to make," said the organisation's CEO Margaret Foti.[12] It was going to take months for them to work out the financial implications of that decision.

Not content with travelling to North America, the disease headed off around the Pacific Rim. One other guest at the Metropole was twenty-six-year-old former flight attendant Esther Mok. She flew home to Singapore and infected twenty people in five days, among them her mother, her father and a pastor who visited her in hospital. All three died, and once again hospital staff and their families were infected.[13] By March 14 there had been 100 cases in Singapore, all of which could ultimately be traced back to Mok, but there was every indication that in this highly controlled country, the authorities were getting the situation under control.

The Chinese Respond

Life in Hong Kong seemed far less certain. On March 27, the department of health announced drastic measures, including vigorous contact tracing and examination, quarantine of contacts in their houses and closure of all schools and universities. A major hospital was designated for infected patients.[14] The move came on the same day that reports from many different parts of China suggested that SARS was spreading within that vast country.

On April 1, and with 685 reported cases and sixteen deaths in Hong Kong alone, the authorities ordered all the residents from Amoy Gardens apartment block to go and stay in a holiday camp – and it wasn't an April Fool's joke, because the SARS virus had taken up residence.[15] The source of this outbreak appeared to be a person who had been treated on ward 8A of the Prince of Wales Hospital because of severe kidney disease and had picked up the bug there. While the treatment was going on, he was staying with his brother at Amoy Gardens.[16]

Remember who else was on ward 8A? Yes, the airport worker who had visited the Metropole. Over the first two weeks of March, fifteen doctors, fifteen nurses, seventeen medical students and five other staff who were associated with that ward became infected and came down with SARS.[17]

Sadly, the kidney patient developed diarrhoea, a symptom that increasingly came to be linked to SARS. In many viral infections, viruses are shed in faeces, and SARS appears to conform. It seems that the infection most probably spread to other residents of Amoy Gardens because the sewers in the complex were leaking, allowing aerosols of virus-containing material to escape into the narrow passageways that ran between the buildings. As if this was not bad enough, sewage also back-flowed into bathroom floor drains in some apartments.[18] Within a matter of days, the estate suddenly had three hundred people who were ill with respiratory problems. It makes little difference building hi-tech hospitals in a city where there are lax attitudes towards basic systems of hygiene.

Living with the Enemy

Anyone who knows anything about 1918 knows that a viral epidemic of a novel virus can have disastrous consequences. The question on everyone's minds was whether these were the birth-pains of the next huge pandemic, or an intriguing and tragic illness that would rapidly run its course and then disappear of its own accord.

As time passed, the WHO became decidedly twitchy. In 1918, the new 'flu was shifted around the world by the mass movement of armies and refugees. In 2003, public transport would do the job very nicely. The WHO decided to try and slow down the flow in some of the more strategic zones. The organisation started by advising that people avoid travelling to Hong Kong and Guangdong unless their trip was of paramount importance. It was a stunning blow, as trade and travel go hand in hand. Up until now, the Chinese authorities had been, at best, reluctant to allow Western agencies into the country, but at the beginning of April, realising that things were getting serious, they invited a WHO team to visit Guangdong.

China is a proud nation with a rich history, and rightly feels that it has a culture that predates that of many countries in the West. It is consequently slow to issue apologies, but on April 4, apologise it did. Speaking at a press conference attended only by local journalists, the director of the Chinese communicable disease control unit said: "Today, we apologise to everyone... Our medical departments and our mass media suffered poor coordination. We weren't able to muster our forces in helping to provide everyone with scientific publicity and allowing the masses to get hold of this sort of knowledge."

A couple of weeks later and the apologies rang out again. This time it was the Chinese Minister of Health who admitted failings over SARS and said that the situation was worse than previously admitted. He was promptly fired, along with the Mayor of Beijing.

Then the clampdown really began in earnest. A correspondent to the *British Medical Journal* described what life was like in China. "I live in Zhejiang, a coastal province halfway between the two Chinese epicentres of the disease, Guangdong and Beijing," wrote Thérèse Hesketh. "Here following the press conference, the government immediately held an emergency meeting. By the next morning a whole raft of measures was in place. All cinemas, theatres, and karaoke bars were closed. All public training courses and meetings and all school outings were cancelled. All buses, trains, taxis, train stations, bus stations, airports were to be disinfected. The May Day holiday was cancelled."[19]

She went on to say that at 7 o'clock the following morning, she was handed a leaflet about SARS prevention at the gate of her compound. It recommended that people wash their hands regularly and warned them about going into crowded places, and described the dangers of nose-picking. The leaflet said that masks would only be effective if they had a minimum of 16 layers and were changed every four hours. When she took her son to school, they found that order was breaking down, as all six hundred children were having their temperatures taken before being allowed into class. It wasn't a one-off. The pupils had their temperatures taken twice a day and anyone with a reading over 38°C was immediately taken to hospital.

According to Hesketh, mass disinfections were set up in the city, and there was a run on masks and thermometers. Supermarkets were soon full of people stocking up on basic essentials and the buses were unusually empty. Where people did need to cram together, such as on aircraft, up to eighty per cent of them wore masks and everyone had to sign a health form before embarking. Temperature scanners were used at airports to check passengers before they took off and after they landed – at times passengers' temperatures were also taken during the flight. People's temperatures were monitored as they arrived at hotels.

Working for a publishing company in China, British national Philip Dorman watched the unfolding events with a mixture of amusement and bemusement. "The initial attempt to keep SARS under wraps was a misguided, but not entirely surprising response," he explained. "The twin party and government structures that run China are well accustomed to misreporting events up the power chain, and the top level were not going to let some 'flu epidemic (which is probably how they would have understood it regardless of what doctors might have told them) in Guangzhou ruin the smoothest transfer of power in post-liberation China. It was only when the doctor from Guangzhou fled to HK and infected a cross-section of people that the truth started to come out and the media got interested."

Consequently, SARS may have played an important part in bringing about political change in China. "Because foreign interest, from media, governments and people like the WHO started to uncover so much of the truth, and there was a lot of unconfirmed speculation beyond that, the Chinese government had to come clean," said Dorman. "Part of that coming-clean process saw a relaxing of media controls and a general increased interest amongst the middle classes here in the business of government. As the central government had to distance itself from those lower down the food chain, whom it blamed for lying to them, so they allowed the media to 'out' these people and to debate how the country is run. After such a period of opening there is always a reactionary adjustment, but some changes have stuck. I guess the best way to sum it all up is as another step in the slow process of China modernising, which will ultimately involve political reform. That reform has to strike a balance between being quick enough for the people, but slow enough to avoid another bloody event like Tiananmen Square, 1989."

If the West thought it had got away with it, then it was time to think again. On April 23, the WHO issued a travel warning that covered not only Beijing and Shanzi Province in China, but also included Toronto. It is only the second time in the fifty-five-year history of the WHO that the organisation has issued a travel advisory, the first being in 1994 when it recommended avoiding travel to parts of India because of plague.

The reaction in Canada was heated. Politicians and scientists queued up at microphones to voice their displeasure. The chief microbiologist at Mount Sinai Hospital, Toronto, accused the WHO of making the travel ban in order to try and appease ruffled feathers in China.[20] All the same, they had to admit that they did have fourteen deaths and three hundred or more suspected cases of SARS in Canada,[21] most of which were in the central province of Ontario. In addition, a forty-six-year-old woman in the Philippines may have contracted the disease in Toronto. The health officials were more cautious in their response. "If we start to see increasing numbers [of cases not linked to hospitals, travel and direct exposure to a SARS case], then I think we're going to have a very great difficulty controlling this outbreak," said Jay Keystone, who worked at the University of Toronto's Centre of Travel and Tropical Medicine. But, he added, "while it's a danger... I don't think we're there yet."

Thankfully, the increase never came. To be considered for a WHO travel advisory, an area must have more than sixty cases of SARS, report more than five new cases daily for an extended period, and show evidence of transmission beyond healthcare workers and their close contacts. With no new cases of people picking up the disease in the community over the previous twenty days, the WHO lifted its travel advice against Toronto on April 30.

Things may have been looking up in Canada, but China was still struggling. By May its tally of cases had risen to 4,280, with 206 people dead. The major centre was now Beijing, which alone had 1,897 cases and 121 deaths. The only good news was that the rate of increase was beginning to decline – things were getting worse more slowly. Likewise, in Taiwan things were looking grim. Over the last couple of weeks of April numbers of cases had tripled, with 116 people infected, and sixteen of them dead. "We suspect that their infection-control measures in hospitals are just not working," commented Peter Cordingly, WHO's spokesman in Manila.[22] It was only a matter of days before the WHO included Taipei, Taiwan, in their list of countries to avoid.

In late May, reports came through that the first case had turned up in the UK, but that the patient seemed to be recovering. Obviously the virus hadn't given up globetrotting.

Health authorities in the United States also started to see people visiting their doctors with symptoms that looked worryingly like SARS. At one point there were 409 suspected cases in forty-two states and Puerto Rico, though this soon narrowed down to eight people who definitely had the disease. Within the previous ten days, seven of these had travelled to areas of the world where the virus was at large in the community. The eighth person was the spouse of someone who had recently returned from Hong Kong and was already confirmed as having SARS.[23]

Just as life in Toronto was getting back into gear, there came another blow. A new outbreak had escaped from the SARS ward on the eighth floor of North York General Hospital. It appears that a ninety-six-year-old man contracted the disease when he went into the hospital on April 19 for surgery for a fractured pelvis. While in the hospital he came down with a chest infection and everyone assumed it was pneumonia – a likely assumption given his age. In fact, he had SARS and died on May 1. Several members of his family, however, soon started to have difficulty breathing and they became part of a new cluster of cases.

In addition, a woman from the hospital's orthopaedic ward who was transferred to St John's Rehabilitation Hospital on April 28 was later recognised as having a mild case of SARS, and five other SARS cases then appeared at St John's Hospital. The woman recovered, one ninety-year-old died, and three others became seriously ill.[24]

As spring turned into summer in the northern hemisphere, the world had witnessed over 6,000 cases, and in some areas industry was feeling the pinch. But there is always a silver lining. The air filtration industry felt that Christmas had come early. Market analysts were predicting that SARS would help fuel an eight per cent year-on-year increase in filter sales as hospitals expanded the number of isolation rooms and improved the filtration of re-circulated air.[25]

The Nature of the Bug

SARS was the first new disease to crop up in the age of genetic technology, and as soon as health officials realised the potential scale of this agent, scientists shot off to their labs to discover what it was.

The initial concept that SARS was caused by some form of yeast was rapidly dismissed once more information was gathered, as too many victims showed no sign of being infected by the yeast organism. The second theory was that it could be a new form of 'flu virus – after all, East Asia is well-known for generating new forms of 'flu. But by mid-March, a team of scientists at the University of Hong Kong had found an unusual virus that appeared to be a member of the Coronaviridae family. This family of viruses includes some that cause common colds in people, but more serious diseases in animals – including severe pneumonia and diarrhoea. The researchers had obtained the virus from samples taken from two different patients, and then, using their findings and some advanced genetic techniques, had detected the same type of virus in forty-five out of fifty suspected SARS patients. Almost as importantly, they had not found this virus in eighty patients who had well-recognised respiratory diseases, nor in 200 blood donors.[26] By mid-April, the WHO had officially named the coronavirus as the guilty party. Thirteen laboratories in ten different countries had all shown that the virus was present in people who exhibited the SARS symptoms. It had been isolated from these people and grown in laboratory cultures, and this cultured virus had been used to infect laboratory animals, showing that the virus was capable of multiplying within this new host.[27]

Shortly afterwards, geneticists had recorded the genetic code built into the molecules of RNA in the centre of each virus. This turns out to be one of the largest sets of genetic instructions in any known RNA-bearing virus. Comparing this information with the genetic sequences in other corona-viruses showed that it was indeed previously unknown, and most probably a close relative of it lives undetected in some wild or domesticated animal. It appears that the outbreak was triggered when the virus learned to jump ship, and left its animal host for life in a human.

Discovering that the coronavirus is critical to SARS does not mean that the earlier suggestion that *Chlamydia pneumoniae* was the agent was totally wrong. It may be that SARS is triggered by the coronavirus, but then *C. pneumoniae*, or one of a number of other bugs moves in for the kill.

The search was on for the source, and investigators scoured Chinese exotic food markets. One group found the virus in six masked palm civets (*Paguma larvata*) and one raccoon dog (*Nyctereutes procyonoides*) in a market in Shenzhen, southern China in May. They also detected antibodies to the virus in a Chinese ferret badger (*Melogale moschata*). All three are sold as delicacies for human consumption in southern China.

Doubts About Diagnosis

Tackling SARS exemplifies all the problems of hitting an unknown moving target. The first is that of trying to recognise patients with the disease as soon as they show up in a healthcare environment. With the World Wide Web up and running, doctors and scientists could "meet" and share information daily without ever having to leave their corner of the world. This meant that they could all have the best available understanding of knowledge that was emerging, without introducing the risks of travelling to see each other, or even posting letters to each other.

Initially the WHO recommended that doctors watch out for people with dry cough and difficulty breathing. The problem with that advice is that a doctor may see people with those symptoms every day, particularly during the winter and none of them may have SARS, so the detection system is very blunt.

As doctors got more experience with SARS patients they started to re-write the recommendations. But these initial symptoms were noted by doctors looking at patients who were in hospital. By definition, they had had the disease for a couple of days. Increasingly, doctors realised that the earlier signs of the disease were more likely to include fever, shivering and muscle ache – the standard symptoms of 'flu.[28] The spectrum of things to look for may have changed, it may even be more accurate, but it is still pretty imprecise.

Inside the body, however, researchers found that conditions were more severe. Almost all sufferers had significant reductions in the numbers of disease-fighting white cells, and in platelets that are vital for a healthy ability to form blood clots. Studying profiles of biochemical factors in the blood, they also found that people who had high concentrations of lactate dehydrogenase, an enzyme that helps the body cope with a lack of oxygen, were least likely to survive the attack.[29]

And looking inside the bodies of people who died of the disease paints a very nasty picture of what this virus achieves. Working near to the first outbreak of the SARS virus in Guangdong, China, Yanqing Ding and his colleagues at the First Military Medical University, Guangzhou – which is in Guangdong Province – showed that the virus causes extensive devastation throughout the body. The main damage was to the lungs, where some areas had collapsed, some parts had extensive bleeding and in other zones tissue had already died. The lining of the lung was breaking down and fluid was leaking into the air spaces. Looking elsewhere, they found that the spleen and lymph glands had large areas of dead tissue. Throughout the body, blood vessels were breaking down, allowing fluid and blood cells to leak into tissues in the heart, lung, liver, kidney, adrenal gland, some areas of the brain and the centre of muscle blocks. Many small veins contained blood clots. Using electron microscopes they discovered clusters of viruses in lung tissue, providing more evidence that the causal agent is a coronavirus. "These findings will be helpful in under-standing the nature of this disease," said Dr Ding.[30]

In the Clear?

By midsummer 2003, things were beginning to look more positive. SARS was becoming significantly less frequent throughout all regions, and seemed to have disappeared from some. It appeared that 2003 was not going to go down in history alongside 1918.

This of course generated two questions that were clearly related to each other. First of all, was the whole episode an example of health-disaster hype? And secondly, are we in the clear?

Answering the first is almost impossible, because you would have to know what would have occurred had there not been widespread clampdowns in travel, confinement of potential carriers of the virus, and rapid action from the WHO and other health organisations. Civil liberty campaigners were quick to raise questions about the quarantine procedures that cities like Hong Kong and Toronto implemented, and to raise eyebrows when Singapore introduced electronic tagging of suspected cases to ensure that they didn't breach their confinement. But it could easily be that this mass action averted a disaster. In this case, accusing health bosses of crying wolf is at best most unkind.

The alternative view is that SARS is a very minor illness on the world stage, and only received publicity because it looked like threatening white middle class people in the west. In reality, fewer than 10,000 people were infected, and under 2,000 died. Compare this with the mass killers of AIDS, malaria and tuberculosis, and it is almost laughable to be concerned at all.

The second question is no easier to answer. In 1918 the 'flu epidemic ended when the virus just stopped infecting people. Why? Nobody knows. In 2003, the drop in SARS infection rates could have been due to this same process, or to the summer. Scientists soon discovered that this coronavirus lives much longer on cool surfaces than on objects that are exposed to warm sunlight. Summer, in effect, brings with it a natural disinfectant. This keeps transmission at bay, but come the winter it is quite possible that we could see a second explosion of activity. Dr Heymann, one of the WHO's senior disease-chasers commented: "We don't know if this disease is seasonal and will decrease this year but come back next year." It was the start of a waiting game.

In many diseases we know that a few individuals become infected with a virus, but never develop symptoms. They are unaware that the killer is on board, but they do shed billions and billions of viral particles as they move around. You only need one of these super spreaders living in a city to have a remarkable effect at re-seeding the disease when environmental conditions become ripe again. In late June 2003, Canadian doctors found just such a person. More may exist undetected. Just because you don't see disease, doesn't mean the bug has gone.

Then you could add the "small world effect" to this equation. This says everybody in the world is linked to everyone else by just six layers of personal links. Consequently, physicists, psychologists and mathematicians who study these linking systems are busy creating mathematical models that attempt to explain the quick spread of SARS and its virus.

With this fear in mind, governments are not turning their backs on the SARS virus. For example, the European Union announced that it would spend nine million Euros on research into SARS prevention. The research would cover, amongst other things, surveillance and control, clinical manifestations including disease transmission, infection control procedures, interventions and vaccines and risk assessment. And spending large sums of money makes sense. Estimates suggest that in 2003 alone, SARS probably knocked one to two percentage points off the previously predicted eight per cent growth in global markets.

Research is important because, unlike the proverbial leopard, viruses can change their spots. By summer 2003, the SARS virus had mutated into two clearly identifiable forms, and there was no reason to believe that this was the end of its transformation. Each mutation, of course, brings with it the fear that the virus will learn another dastardly way of evading human defences. "With SARS on the decline for now, there is a great need to strengthen the SARS control and surveillance system in China," said Dr Henk Bekedam, the WHO's representative to China. "The system now in place grew out of an emergency response and has to be strengthened for the long run," he continued.

Fears were rekindled when in 2004 scientists found the SARS virus in the sweat glands of people killed by the infection. This time Ding's team in China confirmed that the virus gets almost everywhere in the body, causing them to conclude that it was quite capable of being spread via breath, urine or faeces. Now it was clear that just shaking someone's hand, or touching a virus-laden door handle could be all it might take to become infected.[31] "As a result of our work we recommend new infection control measures, which include getting patients to wear gloves, disposable gowns and eye protection in addition to [special] face masks, and to avoid kissing or touching other people," says lead researcher Dr Ding.

At the same time, Dr Inge Hamming and colleagues at University Hospital Groningen in the Netherlands were also trying to unpack some of the biochemical secrets of the SARS virus that made it so successful.[32] They found that SARS locks on to ACE2 receptors, specific protein molecules that are present on cells in many different organs. This enables it to set up an infection in a large number of different places. Many other viruses grab hold of proteins or other markers that are only present in a restricted number of locations around the body, and thus have more limited ability to attack. "Finding where ACE2 is expressed provides a first step in understanding how and where the virus causes the main symptoms of SARS," says lead researcher Dr Harry van Goor.

The Great Escape

All this laboratory attention is great, but it does mean that around the world there are places where the virus is being kept and deliberately farmed for research. The safety procedures around the labs are tight, but it only takes a single momentary lapse in concentration to let the bug out of the bag.

In September 2003, a twenty-seven-year-old research student at Singapore's high security microbiology laboratories in the National University of Singapore fell ill. The laboratory housed samples of the SARS virus, and soon tests indicated that the student might have the virus on board. She had been researching the West Nile virus in a laboratory that was also conducting research using active SARS coronavirus. An investigation into what went wrong concluded that cross-contamination of West Nile virus samples with the SARS virus in the laboratory was the source of infection. Singaporean authorities immediately quarantined twenty-five people who had been living or working with her. The swift action appeared to work and the disease got no further.

A similar situation in Taiwan was not so simple. Again the virus jumped out of a bio-containment research lab, this time using a forty-four-year-old researcher. It appears that on December 5, 2003 he cleared up some contaminated liquid in his lab. He was trying to get to a conference in Singapore and was possibly in a bit of a hurry. Indeed, he travelled to Singapore before coming down with symptoms and returning home. The situation was soon contained and no one else was infected – but it was a close shave.

"This incident illustrates that SARS presents a continuing threat. In the post-epidemic period, the greatest risk from SARS may be through exposure in laboratories where the virus is used or stored," the WHO said in a statement. "For this reason, WHO urges countries to conduct an inventory of laboratories and samples that they hold and to ensure that the correct biosafety procedures are being followed."

On Saturday April 24 2005, the Chinese authorities sealed off a SARS research laboratory in its capital. Again the virus had broken free and was on the loose. It had infected a 26-year-old woman who worked in the lab. This time there was a delay between initial symptoms and action. The nurse, whose surname was Song, had travelled by train from Beijing to her home in Hefei, capital of the province of Anhui, on March 23, but returned to Beijing when she started to develop a fever. The visit had been enough to infect her mother, who died of a respiratory infection on Monday April 19 – six days before the lab was closed. A nurse who had helped the lab worker also became infected. At the peak of the alert 600 people were placed in quarantine.

Counted Out – But...

With no cases showing up in the latter part of 2004 or the first half of 2005, health officials began to breathe more easily. All the indications are that the heavy containment policies employed had paid off. What could so easily have broken out into a global calamity had been contained. Yes, 8,096 people had been recorded as being infected with the disease, and 1,706 had died, but that is a minuscule number compared to the impact of a global 'flu pandemic.

It wasn't long before the carping began, with people asking whether the WHO and other health authorities had "cried wolf" – creating a fuss about nothing. And here we have a classic dilemma. If the authorities don't act and there is a pandemic then they are blamed for incompetence. If they do act and prevent the pandemic, they are accused of creating an unnecessary panic. It comes down to a balance of cost versus risk. You have to weigh up whether the cost caused by the panic is greater than the risk caused by not chasing the disease. One problem here is that many commentators have never thought of – much less experienced – a pandemic, and so think the risk is small. Let's just hope, for all of our sakes, that they are fortunate enough to remain in that state of ignorance.

The question now is at what level to keep up surveillance programs. No people with a disease is not necessarily the same as no infected people. A version of the virus could simply be moving quietly within the population without triggering disease. It could also be sitting within the cells of other animals, waiting for another chance to jump the species gap. Let's hope also that SARS is gone for good – but let's not drop our guard.

CHAPTER 8 - AIDS

The year 1981 started much like any other year, but it ended up being a turning point in the social consciousness of disease. Five men showed up at different Los Angeles hospitals. They didn't know each other but they shared a common enemy. Each had a particular form of pneumonia caused by *Pneumocystis carinii*, a bug that most people encounter, but to which few succumb. Four of them had a fungal infection in their throats and all were infected by cytomegalovirus. The three who were tested had low white blood cell counts, indicative of poorly working immune systems. Then two died.

Two physicians, Michael Gottlieb and Wayne Shandera submitted a short article to the CDC's *Morbidity and Mortality Weekly Report*, in which they outlined the disease and pointed out that all the patients were homosexual. Their conclusion was that this lifestyle could be linked to the disease. Within weeks a second report was published, this time authored by three groups of medics working in New York, San Francisco and Los Angeles. They too had witnessed this unusual spectrum of symptoms in young gay men. As summer rolled into autumn, forty-five men were either dead or severely ill. GRID, or gay-related immuno deficiency, was becoming a recognised syndrome.

Then it started showing up in drug users of either sex, and before long people with haemophilia were coming down with the scourge. Children born to affected women had the disease at birth. This was not just a gay disease and the title switched to AIDS – acquired immune deficiency syndrome – but it wasn't until 1986 that the causal agent was tracked down and named Human Immunodeficiency Virus (HIV). This was eventually recognised as a lentivirus, a subgroup of a recently discovered group of viruses called retroviruses that have a mechanism for burying themselves within the host cell's chromosomes.

A race was on to be the first person to identify the cause of this perplexing condition. In 1983 Professor Luc Montagnier, Françoise Barré, Jean-Claude Chermann and colleagues at the Pasteur Institute in Paris identified a retrovirus in blood taken from a man who had infected lymph nodes and a condition that doctors thought might be associated with AIDS. They named it LAV – Lymphadenopathy-Associated Virus. At about the same time, a team in San Francisco led by Jay Levy found a similar virus and called their discovery ARV (AIDS-Related Virus).[1] Not only did they find the virus in sick people, but they also identified it in gay men in the San Francisco area who had no symptoms of the disease, for the first time indicating the possibility that people could act as carriers of the disease.

Soon afterward Professor Robert Gallo's team at the National Institute of Health, Bethesda, claimed to have found yet another virus, calling this one HTLV-III (Human T-Cell Lymphotropic Virus III). Their paper said that they found the virus in blood from one US patient and two French patients. Montagnier's and Gallo's observations were published in two separate papers in the same 1983 edition of the journal *Science*.[2,3] A few years later an unholy row broke out about who actually got to the top of this particular mountain first. The catalyst to the dispute was Gallo's application for a patent to cover the test he had developed for detecting HIV. Evidence indicated that the viruses that Gallo claimed to have isolated were in fact none other than those that came from the samples he had been sent by Montagnier. A subcommittee of the US House of Representatives concluded, "There is no longer any doubt that the IP [Institut Pasteur] scientists were first to isolate the AIDS virus. The LTCB [Gallo's Laboratory of Tumour Cell Biology] scientists eventually did isolate and grow their own AIDS viruses; however, they did not discover the AIDS virus isolate with which they performed all of their seminal experiments. Instead they performed all of these experiments with the IP virus, first under its own original name (LAV), then under two different names – MOV and HTLV-IIIb."[4] While Gallo was officially cleared of fraud, a report by the US Office of Research Integrity accused him of "irresponsible laboratory management" and said that the whole episode was a tragedy for science. The story of this hunt shows how easily science can become complicated by the scientists' egos and the passionate desire to claim patents.

It didn't take long before these three viruses were all found to belong to the same group of retroviruses, but were clearly distinct from any that had been seen before. In 1986 the International Committee on Taxonomy of Viruses recommended giving the AIDS virus a separate name – and the initials HIV entered the popular vocabulary.

The search then went global and HIV turned up everywhere researchers looked. They also began to realise that it could lie dormant in a person for the best part of twenty years. Before long it was apparent that there were two clear types of the agent, one that was prevalent in the US and Europe (dubbed HIV-1) and the other in West Africa (HIV-2). Both sub-types cause AIDS, but compared with HIV-1, HIV-2 seems to be less capable of causing disease and less efficiently transferred between adults and children.

HIV infection and AIDS have since become pandemic with over thirty-four million people estimated to be infected in the year 2000 and just under three million deaths per year.

What Is HIV-AIDS?

AIDS crept up on an unsuspecting medical profession. Two decades later much more is known about the disease, but it seems to exists in shadows, as there is much still to discover. There is even dissent about the actual cause of the disease. South African President Thabo Mbeki famously caused a storm by declaring that science had got it wrong. In his opinion, AIDS was not caused by HIV, but by poverty, malnutrition, poor hygiene and local diseases.

In an effort to rebut what they thought was a dangerous misunder-standing, scientists took an unprecedented step. Just before an international AIDS convention opened in Durban, South Africa, in July 2000, some five thousand scientists from fifty countries signed a declaration. Published in the July 6, 2000 edition of *Nature*, it was unequivocal. "HIV causes AIDS. It is unfortunate that a few vocal people continue to deny the evidence. This position will cost countless lives," was its take-home message. "In this global emergency, prevention of HIV infection must be our greatest worldwide public health priority. The knowledge and tools to prevent infection are available... But to tackle the disease, everyone must first understand that HIV is the enemy...". Towards the end, the declaration starts to sound a little more like a preacher proclaiming the religion of science. "There is no end in sight to the AIDS pandemic. But, by working together, we have the power to reverse its tide. Science will one day triumph over AIDS, just as it did over smallpox...".

Let's see what we do know about the disease. The virus moves about in body fluids. Thankfully it can't be coughed or sneezed into the air. It can move into a developing baby by crossing the placenta and entering the baby's blood stream. It is also very successful at passing from one person to another during sexual intercourse, particularly anal sex. Sharing contaminated needles with a person who has HIV in their blood stream is another way of picking it up, and HIV-AIDS is particularly prevalent among drug users. Before 1985 many people with haemophilia became infected via infusions of the blood-clotting factor that they need to treat their illness. People with HIV had given blood and the virus had passed into the medicine. HIV has been isolated from lymphocytes in peripheral blood, cell-free plasma, semen, cervical secretions, cerebrospinal fluid, tears, saliva, urine and breast milk.

The Nature of the Beast

Like many viruses, HIV is spherical, but at about 0.1 microns in diameter, it is small even for a virus. The outer surface or coat has seventy-two spike-like molecules constructed of glycoproteins gp120 and gp42. These spikes are important in the way that the virus causes disease. Like the 'flu virus, the whole unit looks much like a floating mine. Or at least it does when it pops out of a cell as a newly born virus. Some electron-microscopic observations suggest that the spikes fall off rapidly.

Inside the spherical coat is a cone-shaped core, or capsid. This, like the nucleus of many cells, contains its genetic information. HIV is an RNA virus in which the genes are stored in duplicate on two virtually identical strands of RNA. On these two threadlike molecules, the virus stores information to build just two structural proteins, three enzymes and six other proteins that regulate the virus' replication. That's all the information needed to devastate whole communities and bring nations to their knees.

A critical aspect of successful infection is breaking into a cell. The cells favoured by HIV are T-helper cells, a type of white blood cells that plays a key role in a human being's immune system. The surface of these cells are studded with CD4 molecules, proteins that are remarkably capable of locking on to HIV's gp120s. The most obvious assumption is that the affinity between gp120 and CD4 locks the virus to the T-helper cell allowing the cell to swallow the virus. It's a great theory and may well be true, but it has been complicated by the realisation that the gp120 molecules can be shed rapidly by the virus. Could it be that only very young viruses use this mechanism, and older ones have another mode of action? Time, and research, will tell.

T-helper cells are designed to fight viruses, so any cell that swallows a virus would have thought that it had done a good job. Now, however, things go wrong. Inside the cell the virus avoids destruction. Instead, reverse transcriptase copies its RNA to DNA. This DNA then enters the cell's nucleus and becomes spliced into one of the chromosomes.

There is also some evidence that the gp120 studs on the outside of the virus act as molecular camouflage because they mimic molecules that the immune system is used to coming across. Their presence appears to mess up the immune system's highly regimented processes. This could be one reason why the virus can hang around in a person for so long without being evicted.

Reverse transcriptase is packaged along with the RNA in the capsid. Once the virus has penetrated a T-helper cell this enzyme takes the RNA and builds a DNA replica, a provirus, that contains the virus' genetic code. This DNA replica then moves from the cytoplasm into the cell's nucleus and becomes incorporated into its chromosomes. It is a remarkable process, because it is the reverse of what normally happens. Animal cells only have enzymes that allow the nucleus-contained DNA to be transcribed into RNA and this RNA then travels from the nucleus to the cytoplasm. The presence of this enzyme is the origin of the name retrovirus, because it allows the information on the RNA to move in a retrograde direction.

Once incorporated into the host cell's chromosome the provirus may lie dormant in the host cell DNA, thus forming a "latent" infection of the cell. In this state no virus particles are produced and the immune system has no way of spotting that the cell is infected, so it leaves the cell unmolested.

The cell continues to function normally until something triggers the provirus into action. The nature of the trigger is poorly understood – it is an area of more theories than facts. If, in the meantime, the cell divides, the information is copied into the two new cells. It's a sneaky way of extending the scope of the infection.

At some time in the future, this DNA instructs the building of new RNA which moves back from the nucleus into the main body of the cell and sets to work ordering the cell to start building new viral proteins immediately. Some of these proteins, including gp120, become incorporated into the T-helper cell's membrane. When the contents of the virus have been assembled the new virus escapes the cell by budding off and taking a section of glycoprotein-studded host cell membrane with it. Therefore the new virus has its identifying glycoproteins ready built-in.

There are many puzzles still to be resolved. One is that the proportion of T-helper cells infected with HIV is very small, too small to account for the level of T-cell loss. One theory suggests that the infected T-cells are quickly spotted by other players in the body's immune system and destroyed. New cells then replace them. The total number of T-cells declines when the body's system for producing them becomes exhausted. The theory is not complete, because it fails to explain why it takes more than a decade for the decline in T-cells to become catastrophic.

During the first few weeks following infection by HIV the virus replicates rapidly and there are loads of them floating around in the blood. The virus gets everywhere and the person may feel as if they have mild 'flu. The effect is so mild that many don't even notice it. This initial phase is followed by a decrease in the concentration of virus in the blood and a symptom-free period. In the background, however, the virus is continuing to replicate and deplete the immune cells and moving into and damaging lymph nodes. Symptoms only appear after this has been going on for around ten years.

The term AIDS is only used when the person starts to suffer from a range of different infections or tumours that have the opportunity of moving in because his or her immune system is at such a low ebb. As this is slightly arbitrary, epidemiologists studying the incidence and spread of the disease use a definition based on HIV infection and the number of T-cells – if the person has HIV and less than two hundred cells per microlitre of blood, they are classified as having AIDS.

As the white cell count falls, the person's immune system gets progressively weaker and the subject becomes susceptible to less and less virulent pathogens. This means that they can fall prey to many other infections that normally they would have fought off, such as tuberculosis, oral thrush, long-lasting gut infections and pneumonia. Some people under the age of sixty also succumb to a particular form of skin cancer called Kaposi's Sarcoma. Cytomegalovirus infection, which does nothing to healthy people, can get into an HIV patient's retina, scarring the delicate and previously transparent sheet of cells, and resulting in blindness.

It's notoriously difficult to predict how long an individual person will survive once symptoms have broken out, but two years makes a good estimate, though this is highly dependent upon which opportunistic infections the person encounters.

Why is HIV So Deadly?

HIV has five key strategies that have made it one of the most remarkably successful disease-causing viruses. It hides, it mutates slowly, it has sex and it is a shy subversive. Finally, the trump card, it is transmitted by sex and drug abuse.

An Undercover Subversive

Retroviruses' ingenious trick of burying their DNA in the host cell's genome holds one key to AIDS success. It can sit there silently lying dormant for just as long as it likes. Because it is effectively inactive the host cell is not targeted by the immune system and carries on its duties as if nothing has happened. The genome therefore represents a hiding place for the virus and even if the body mounts a huge immune response it cannot eliminate all proviruses. If the virus infects the cells that build new T-cells and integrate themselves into that genome, then every new T-cell manufactured comes with its very own virus already built in.

If germ cells in the testes or ovaries, which produce sperm and eggs, become infected, retroviruses may be passed down the generations. As a result, some retroviruses have been present in certain species so long that they are now considered part of the species' genome.

Minor Mutations

But that's not the only trick that HIV has. When proviral DNA is transcribed back into RNA they have another opportunity to cause chaos. The rate of production of new RNA is rapid. Thousands, millions, maybe even billions of new strands of RNA are generated. Howard Temin, the scientist who discovered retroviruses called it a "viral swarm". Little surprise then that with production on such a mass scale the odd mistake slips in. The RNA codes have minor differences prompting Nobel Prize winner Manfred Eigen to refer to the resulting viral population as a "quasi-species".

Each change is minor and the effect can't be predicted. Most will have little effect, some will render the virus impotent. Just a few changes will make it more lethal or more capable of evading detection by the immune system. Such diversity affords the virus unprecedented flexibility and resilience to changes in the environment. Those that survive will be much fitter and more formidable. It's basically the principle of Darwinian natural selection played out at high speed, and is a key to HIV's success.

Antigenic variation is the name of the game. The white cells of the body's immune system constantly search around, looking in every nook and cranny for unwelcome squatters. Is it friend or foe – part of the family or a foreigner? Their method is to scrutinise the surface of any cell or particle that they encounter, checking that it recognises all of the molecules. Some cells are trained like sniffer-dogs to search out specific individual villains. These are the types of cells that are boosted by vaccination and they look for recognised antigens, identifiable features of the surface that occur on invading particles or organisms. With HIV, the immune system searches the virus' surface checking out its proteins to see whether any of them have been associated with an intruder before. By constantly mutating its genes, HIV alters the nature of these protein antigens, so that trying to combat HIV is much like trying to hit a moving target.

There are two types of antigenic variation, confusingly known as antigenic drift and antigenic shift.

Antigenic drift is a gradual process. Each new generation of virus has only a couple of mutations throughout its genes. The difference between one generation and the next may be very minor, but it could confer a selective advantage by enabling the virus to avoid immune attack. This type of variation is responsible for epidemics of influenza, where the population has only partial immunity to the virus.

Compared to most biological entities that use DNA or RNA, retroviruses have an unusually high incidence of mutations. The reason for this is that the enzyme they use to transcribe the RNA to DNA, reverse transcriptase, has no error correcting function. Most other systems have exonuclease, an editing enzyme that checks that the code has been faithfully copied and corrects any mistakes. The result is that antigenic drift errors occur at a rate of one change in two thousand to four thousand nucleotides for every generation of virus – many orders of magnitude higher than in human gene replication.

The major source of variation, however, results from antigenic shift, a phenomenon that Temin dubbed "retroviral sex". This sex in a T-cell can have a dramatic effect. In animals and plants, sex is important because it stirs up the gene pool and produces variation. Similarly retroviral sex induces dramatic changes by shuffling large sections of the virus' genome.

HIV has two strands of RNA. In a standard virus, both are identical. But within a population of viruses the strands they carry will have altered slowly due to antigenic drift. Retroviral sex is a two-stage process. The first occurs when two viruses of different strains infect the same cell. Both are transcribed to DNA and both head off into the nucleus. When replication starts the two different strands of RNA are sent into the body of the cell and pairs form at random. Some of the pairs will be from the same initial strain, but some will have one strand that came from one strain, and the second strand from the other. The new virus will acquire mutations that have accumulated in two different branches of HIV's genealogical tree.

Stage two occurs when this heterozygous virus containing dissimilar RNA strands infects a new cell. Now, during the transcription process, the two strands are shuffled. Offspring viruses that bud from this cell will again have identical, homozygous, strands of RNA, but they will be a mosaic of the two sets of genes that were present in the original two strains.

Antigenic shift causes pandemics because the population has no acquired immunity to the virus. Until the emergence of HIV, influenza represented the last great pandemic disease.

The Waiting Game

Years pass between the a person's initial infection and the first clear symptoms of disease. This enabled the virus to spread far and wide before anyone starts looking for it. Gaetan Dugas, a Canadian air steward famously became branded with the title Patient Zero. It's a term epidemiologists give to the first person who got a disease and the central character in an epidemic outburst. Dugas was gay and claimed that he had sexual relations with two hundred and fifty men a year. In all he says that he probably had two and a half thousand sexual partners. In *And The Band Played On*, Randy Shilts describes how Dugas refused to curb his sexual behaviour even after doctors told him that he could be passing on the disease to others: "Someone gave this thing to me. I'm not going to give up sex."[5] He died on March 30, 1984.

It now seems most unlikely that Dugas was a true Patient Zero, in that AIDS probably had many more than one entry point into America, and has a much more complex pattern of spread around the world than could be explained by the one man. It was only in the last months of his life that Dugas, like many others, realised that they had a transmissible disease and by the time he knew it vast damage had already been done.

The long symptom-free period also gives HIV plenty of time to mutate, so that after a ten-year infection, a person will be inhabited by a mixture of variant types of HIV. In reality, it is unlikely that a person is infected by a single strain in the first place, because the virus had almost certainly mutated in the previous sufferer.

This poses huge problems both for research and for treatment. In both situations you want to collect blood from an individual and see what mutants of the virus are present. Different mutants, however, grow at different rates in the body and in a laboratory culture system. The particular mutant that is doing most damage and is present in largest numbers in the patient may not thrive in the laboratory and can be overshadowed by other mutants. Consequently, it's very difficult for doctors to know the exact nature of the virus in any individual patient.

This uncertainty hinders therapy. How can you target drugs, or give accurate prognoses, if you are uncertain of the precise set of mutations present in one person's HIV? Added to this is the probability that an individual is carrying many different mutations, each of which will have slightly different responses to specific drug therapies.

Adding these four manoeuvres together means that HIV inevitably adapts to resist anti-viral chemotherapy. Any therapy thrown at it will wipe out vast numbers of the viruses, but there is always likely to be one or two mutants that find a loophole. That mutation will be untouched and live on, maintaining the disease. The result is that all drugs in current use have a limited time during which they are effective.

The Ace of Spades

The sexual revolution had changed the world. In western societies, the old order where everyone had to stick to one partner of the opposite sex, or pretend that this was what they were doing, had been swept aside. Women had made the first steps in being set free from the social shackles that kept them as objects of male desire and useful things to keep around the house. Flower power, contraceptive pills and recreational sex seemingly were now going along hand in hand. Homosexuality was gaining ever-increasing acceptance. The social order, or rather disorder, in the continent of Africa helped fuel the fire. Work practices meant that men travelled hundreds of miles to work on farms and mines, returning only occasionally to their families. While away they were entertained in brothels. Back at home they introduced the disease to their villages and townships.

Whatever you think of free sex, it certainly gave HIV a free ride. The newly emerging order was, and in many places still is, a perfect environment for AIDS to flourish. The uncomfortable truth suddenly dawned. Sexual intercourse is an effective way of transferring HIV. In heterosexual and homosexual sex, the receptive partner of the sexual act is always at most risk. If a man is infected, HIV will be present in semen and this finds easy passage through the vaginal or bowel wall, but HIV also infects the walls of the bowel and vagina so infections can pass in either direction. There is a two- to five-fold greater risk of the infection moving from male to female than from female to male. Female-to-male transmission does, however, increase if the sex act coincides with the woman's period. Transmission rates seem to have more to do with the number of partners a person has, rather than the frequency of sex with a single partner, and homosexual sex seems to be more efficient at passing on the bug than does heterosexual sex.

A few years ago I visited an AIDS education centre in the south of Zimbabwe where female sex workers were being trained to spread the message. It was shocking to see these women practising songs and street theatre that they would later perform in marketplaces and brothels, knowing that most of them must be infected with HIV and all would probably die at its behest. The centre's message was simple: safe sex is abstinence, or, failing that, use a condom.

But how good are condoms? In 1992 the FDA released data from a study that appeared to show that HIV could penetrate condoms.[6] Not surprisingly, this caused grave concern. The researchers had set up an artificial system and found that fluorescent glass beads of about the size of a virus particle could leak through a latex condom. They did point out that even given their data you were much safer wearing a condom than throwing them away, but you were still at risk. The CDC, however, took issue with this work and issued a fact sheet pointing to flaws in the FDA's work and saying that a correctly used condom gives very good protection.[7] Condoms, however, are no good if they are damaged or too old.

Where Does HIV Come From?

This begs the question though — where did HIV start? Promiscuity, drug use and blood transfusion have certainly served to propagate it at an alarming rate, but this doesn't help to identify its origins. If anything, the rate of its spread makes that task harder.

Edward Hooper starts his epic thousand-page book *The River* by listing the various possibilities that have been proposed — some weird, some wacky, some plausible. They include the idea that "AIDS came from God, and it punished homosexuals, junkies, and other perverts and reprobates. Or it came from a man, who was aiming at roughly the same groups that God was after. It came from outer space, on the tail of a comet. It came from Africa, through people eating monkeys. It came from Africa, through kinky stuff with monkeys. It came from Haiti, and had something to do with swine fever and voodoo rites. It came from scientists, from hepatitis B, or smallpox, or polio vaccine gone wrong. It had always been around, but had escaped only recently from the confines of an isolated tribe. It had always been with us, and was merely syphilis, malnutrition, TB, the effects of hard drugs — or combinations of the above — lumped together and given a new name."[8] There's also the theory that it was a man-made biological weapon that got out of control.

As the dust settles, a consensus is appearing. HIV came from African apes. HIV-2 was the first to be located, and that turns out to have come from the West African sooty mangabey monkey (*Cercocebus atys*) and HIV-1 from *Pan troglodytes troglodytes*, a sub-species of chimpanzee, that lives in the Central African rainforest.[9] Both of these animals carry a remarkably similar virus, Simian Immunodeficiency Virus (SIV). The animals do not get ill, which suggests that they and their forebears have lived with the virus for long enough to develop a natural immunity to it.

This much is now fairly uncontentious. The problem is deciding how the virus hopped ship and moved to human beings. The traditional line is that a hunter with a sore mouth ate some poorly cooked ape meat, picked up the virus and passed it on. It's a reasonable theory and there are plenty of monkeys and chimpanzees killed and eaten each year. But this has been going on for as long as humans have lived near monkeys, and the virus seems to have been in monkeys for ages, so why wait until the 1950s before making the change? Now the standard theory looks to social trends and politics, claiming that the infection had often crossed over, but it was only in the 1950s that promiscuity and labour practices combined to give HIV an ideal breeding ground. The flaws in this argument are that the socio-political changes happened earlier, that sexual promiscuity is not a new phenomenon and that no case of HIV infection came to America in any of the ten million men, women and children exported by the slave-trade. HIV-AIDS must be a new disease that started life in and around the 1950s.

In *The River*, Hooper presents evidence suggesting that the explosion of cases came from HIV-infected batches of polio vaccine that were given to a million people in the former Belgian Congo and regions of Rwanda-Burundi between February 1957 and June 1960, nicely in time for the mid-1970's pandemic. Parts of the Congo that received the vaccine had a high incidence of early cases of AIDS. Parts that did not receive the vaccine had no cases. Hooper's book created quite a stir. Hooper says that he is not interested in recrimination, only in searching after the truth, but you can easily see that a few lawyers might see things a little differently.

Hooper spent nine years stacking up the evidence and he has left few stones unturned. He maintains that Hilary Koprowski of the Wistar Institute in Philadelphia developed the polio vaccine by growing viruses on kidneys taken from African chimpanzees. The vaccine became known as CHAT, but the interpretation of the acronym seems uncertain. One possibility is that it stands for "Chimpanzee Adapted and Tested". Koprowski denies any link between the vaccine and chimpanzees, but he is unable to give a convincing account of what species of primate the kidneys did come from. Certainly, chimpanzee kidneys were flown to Philadelphia at about the right time and white blood cells carrying SIV are quite capable of hiding in kidneys.

One argument against this theory was that a man from Manchester, England, apparently died from AIDS in 1959. When stored samples from this person were re-examined, however, no trace of HIV was found – a case of mistaken identity. All other cases of people outside Africa who had AIDS in the 1960s and early 1970s had direct links with the area where the polio vaccine was given. This even included the first known American case, a 16-year-old mother who gave birth to an HIV-positive child in 1973 or 1974. It turns out that as a baby, this woman was with her mother in a New Jersey women's prison at the time when babies were given the first trial batches of polio vaccine.

The implications were shocking. A mass rush to rid the world of one scourge had unleashed another. The final test of Hooper's theory would be to carry out tests on the few remaining vials of CHAT. If HIV was found in the vaccine the story would be concluded. If it wasn't it would only prove that those vials were free of the disease – other batches could have been infected.

November 2000 saw this story turn another corner. After years of saying there were no original vials of CHAT vaccine, one was suddenly discovered and offered for testing. Four different research groups analysed the contents and each failed to find any sign of the HIV virus. The result was a massive press assault to discredit Hooper and his book. Koprowski suggested that Hooper's publisher was, perhaps, more interested in sensationalism than truth, resulting in the publication of a book that was totally erroneous. On April 26, 2001, the science journal *Nature* ran an article entitled "The River without a paddle", which stated that Hooper's claim had been dealt what could be a fatal blow.

If anyone expected Hooper to put his hands up and say that he was wrong, they were to be disappointed. Speaking at a hastily arranged meeting at the Royal Society in London, UK, Hooper pointed to a series of flaws in this latest research, each of which raised questions about these findings. The scientists then fired back counter-claims, airing their theories in a series of press releases.

One of the problems at the end of the day is that science is not good at proving or disproving things beyond all doubt. "It is the old problem of proving a negative," said Neil Berry of the National Institute for Biological Standards and Control. But the data really doesn't provide any support for his hypothesis.

Another problem is that science stands to lose credibility if this theory is allowed to stand, and there is a strong vested interest in seeing its downfall, even if there is no conclusive evidence to disprove it.

And the lessons? One is that finding the origins of a new disease will never be easy and may normally be impossible. The detective work is not simple and is seldom irrefutable. On top of this, evidence can easily be distorted either intentionally or unwittingly by those who stand to rise or fall depending on the results of an investigation. Did HIV-AIDS come from a tragic error in the polio programme? The highest possibility is that we will almost certainly never know for certain, but the fact remains that even if it didn't, it was a possibility.

Another lesson is that using cells from other animals carries dangers. It might not have occured in the case of HIV-AIDS, who knows, but the distinct possibility that it could have was enough to send scores of scientists scurrying around looking at the evidence. The problem is that hidden in animal cells are the geonomes of retroviruses that the animal has learned to live with, but if placed in a new environment these killer genes could break out and recreate their viruses generating unforseen consequences.

Rigorous testing is vital. At the moment there is a branch of medical science developing ways of genetically modifying pigs so that their organs will avoid detection by a human immune system. A major centre of this work is in Babraham just outside Cambridge, England. They could then become a valuable source of donor organs – hearts, kidneys, lungs, etc. Such xeno-transplantation does, however, carry a frightful risk. Retroviruses could move from pigs to humans. "The likelihood of this occurring is probably impossible to predict. However, xenotransplantation produces the most wonderful culture system for totally new viruses to arise," says the director of the Institute of Virology and Environmental Microbiology, Pat Nuttall. "It is possible that viruses from different species might be placed in an environment that removes all the selective pressures that normally prevent survival. It is conceivable that this could generate a virus that has never been experienced by humans, with potentially disastrous consequences."[10]

Cocktail Bar

Once you have HIV on board, it will be there for the rest of your life. There is no known way of driving it out. The best that medicine can offer is a cocktail of three different drugs costing in the order of £10,000/$14,000 per year. AZT (zidovudine) is the best known name in HIV therapy. It's a chemical that looks a lot like thymidine, one of the building blocks of DNA, and it prevents the viral RNA being transcribed when the virus breaks into a cell. The problem is that it also disrupts the DNA inside mitochondria, the cell's power stations, leading to symptoms that include insomnia, fever, headaches, confusion and anxiety depression. Still, it does reduce the numbers of viruses floating around in a person's blood and helps stave off some of the opportunistic infections that are so damaging.

Add to AZT a couple of new entrants to the pharmaceutical bar, and the triple therapy is more powerful. Protease inhibitors are the current boy-wonders, and Invirase is a front runner. These block the viruses' ability to break out of their host cell. There are a dozen or so possible drugs to choose from. They can all have unpleasant side effects and they are all expensive and even then triple therapy won't stop the disease — it simply has the possibility of slowing it down or increasing the amount of symptom-free time.

Attempts to produce a vaccine have been thwarted by the pace at which HIV changes. Just as soon as you have a vaccine that targets the virus, the virus mutates. Time to build a new vaccine. Most vaccines start life as the disease-causing virus that is then weakened, by exposing it to either chemical or physical assault. Unfortunately, no-one has found a way of weakening AIDS. The live vaccines that have been tested in labs have a tendency to induce cancer — not good. Breaking the virus to pieces and just using the bits of protein works for other viruses, but not for AIDS as it fails to stimulate the immune system.

The best hope appears to come from newly-emerging genetic technologies. Genetic vaccines offer exciting possibilities to combat many diseases, and HIV-AIDS could fall under their spell. The idea with a vaccine is that you give a bit of the disease and the body remembers what it looks like so that it can fight it in the future. With a genetic vaccine you take one or two genes that produce specific proteins within the disease-causing agent. Injecting this genetic material into body cells causes the cells to produce this protein. The body's immune system spots this foreign protein and reacts against it. A class of memory cells then comes into being that spends its life looking for other examples of this material. When the disease-causing agent shows up the immune system is ready and waiting. Scientists working in this area have levelled their sights on a variety of diseases — herpes, influenza, hepatitis B and HIV — but it will still take years to develop the vaccine and more years to test that it is safe.

Another genetically based technique makes ingenious use of one process that is unique to the virus. HIV uses the enzyme protease as a pair of biological scissors, and employs it to snip its way out of the cell that has just built it. A group of researchers at the Washington University School of Medicine have built TAT-Casp3, a novel protein that these scissors can easily cut in half. When whole, the new protein is inert, but the TAT element allows it to slip through cell membranes. When cut in half, the TAT section is removed and the Casp3 piece becomes active. This is a human enzyme, which causes the cells containing it to commit suicide. The protein can get into any cells, but only cells infected with HIV have the protease needed to activate it, so only disease-bearing cells die.[11] The leader of the research, Steven Dowdy, believes that this Trojan horse could be used to combat many other infectious diseases, such as hepatitis C, malaria and herpes.

After a decade or more of research, scientists know a great deal about why vaccines won't work, but still have to come up with some truly successful alternatives. It's safe to say that there's no HIV vaccine just over the horizon.

Future

The immediate future looks grim. At the start of the new millennium HIV has a massive grip on Africa. Up to one third of all people living in Botswana are infected, as are a quarter of the people in Lesotho, Swaziland and Zimbabwe and a fifth of those in Namibia and Zambia. One in twenty people living in the Bahamas and Haiti have HIV. The incidence in India is below one per cent, but with her huge population that still means that over three and a half million people are infected, a total only beaten by South Africa's 4.1 million people with HIV.

By 2003 Botswana, South Africa, and Zimbabwe were experiencing negative population growth, and five other countries in Africa were experiencing a growth rate of nearly zero. "Not since the Black Death devastated medieval Europe has humankind observed infectious disease deaths on such a massive scale that a country's population has shrunk rather than grown. But that scenario is playing out again in the twenty-first century, with HIV/AIDS replacing bubonic plague as the killer," comments HIV expert Joan Stephenson.[12]

Infection rates in the West dropped in the 1990s, and this has led to an ominous culture of complacency in many western countries. Ominous because there is little sign of the infection rate going down anywhere else. In fact, in many countries AIDS is just making its first advances into the unsuspecting population. There is a desperate need for good information to get to all the people – and fast.

Few other diseases have drawn our attention so strongly to the links between human behaviour, health and infection. This can be seen clearly in a 2005 document published by UNAIDS, and entitled *AIDS in Africa: Three scenarios to 2025*. In this report the authors start by assessing what they call the five key driving forces behind Africa's AIDS epidemics. While summarising them here, it is worth noting that although this exercise focused on AIDS in Africa, the results have much wider application.

The first driving force is the growth or erosion of unity and integration. Societies that live well together will be in a position to implement good healthcare practices, and these will include policies that can control AIDS. If there is violence or conflict, inequality or ethnic and religious tension, then the united effort grinds to a halt. Secondly, having the correct beliefs about how a disease spreads is vital. Societies that give people with the disease a social stigma often make life worse, because the very people who need help in order to take the disease out of society are the people least likely to receive it.

Thirdly, making best use of limited resources and skills is a vital part of the process. The problem is that poor management, corruption, underdevelopment or the sheer scale of the epidemic so often stretch these. The fourth force is the generation and application of knowledge. Science has come a long way in understanding AIDS and in making sense of the link between the disease and particular lifestyles and patterns of sexual behaviour. The task now is to use this knowledge to push for improved chances of having a healthy life.

Finally, the UNAIDS document says that the distribution of power and authority plays a role. Whether power is monopolised or shared can determine the extent of inequality. While the issue is important, there are no quick fixes, as the effect of any political or power system will vary in different cultures.

There is a huge task facing anyone involved in tackling this epidemic, but one thing that we can be thankful for is that AIDS has never mutated into a form that can transmit by any other means than within body fluids. Let's hope it never finds a way of getting into the lungs and then moving on in aerosols as an infected person coughs. But the longer the pandemic goes on, the more chances HIV has of learning new tricks. It's in everybody's interest to stamp out this blight before it gets any worse.

CHAPTER 9 –
. . . AND THEN YOU DISSOLVE

When it comes to infectious diseases, the prizes for gothic horror must go to the haemorrhagic viruses and flesh-eating bacteria. If viruses like Marburg, Ebola, Dengue, Machupo and Lassa, and bacteria such as group A *Streptococcus pneumoni*, don't send a shiver down your spine, then you don't know anything about the suffering they can inflict. There is something deeply disturbing about diseases that cause a person's eyes to turn bright red and their insides to dissolve and erupt in a blood-filled foam from their mouth, nose and anus. The terror is magnified by the uncertainties that surround these outbreaks of medical hell. Is this a virus that we've seen before and know how to contain? Is it a new variant capable of moving from person to person in unexpected ways? Is this type of bacteria going to respond to our antibiotics?

On the Prowl

Dengue haemorrhagic fever is spreading like wildfire. Before 1970 only nine countries had recorded incidences of epidemics. By 1995 that number had risen to around forty. In 1998 it was endemic in one hundred countries in Africa, the Americas, the Eastern Mediterranean, South-East Asia and the Western Pacific. These are highly populated regions, so two-fifths of the world's population are now exposed to this viral disease, with fifty million cases of dengue infection each year.[1]

Thankfully, not all cases of dengue infection progress through to haemorrhagic fever. Of the 616,000 cases of dengue in the Americas in 1998, only eleven thousand had the full-blown disease. But that's a shockingly high number, and it is double the recorded incidence in 1995. Between 1984 and 1993 Mexico had only twenty-six cases, but this rose to thirty in 1994 and then to 358 in 1995. In Brazil in 1998 nearly 475,000 cases of dengue infection were reported, which is more than occurred for the entire continent in previous years. Around the world, about five per cent of people with dengue haemorrhagic fever die. This is a balance between the twenty per cent mortality that occurs if there is no intensive medical support therapy, and the one per cent that can be achieved with the best that modern medicine can supply.

Once again, *Aedes aegypti* is the agent provocateur and the increased incidence of disease is attributed to expanding urban sprawls in which the mosquito finds a comfortable home. Non-biodegradable plastic packaging and discarded tyres are key culprits. They provide shaded water-filled hollows that mosquitoes love to use for laying their eggs and in which their larvae can develop in peace. The virus perpetuates its presence either by moving to a new victim when infected female insects feed, or by getting a transfer to the next generation of insects by stowing away in eggs.

Dengue fever starts as a 'flu-like illness. Young children run a temperature and get a rash. Older children and adults may get headaches, pain behind the eyes and muscle aches. It goes away after a few days and seldom does any serious damage. The illness may last ten days – recovery takes weeks. Dengue haemorrhagic fever is another story. This starts as any normal infection, but the virus just doesn't seem to know when to give in. The liver enlarges and the person's temperature soars to 40–41°C and stays there for two or three days. If they are lucky the symptoms slowly go away. Otherwise they go into a state of shock and die within twelve to twenty-four hours.

There is no particularly good treatment other than trying to manage the patient's blood volume in an intensive care facility. There is no vaccine. If New Yorkers are worried about the West Nile outbreak that started in 1999 (see Chapter 12), they should be petrified about dengue.

In the News

Ebola and its close sister Marburg are viruses that have captured people's imaginations, partly because they are vicious diseases for which we have no cure and also because the stories of their discovery have been told dramatically in a couple of well-written best sellers. Ebola was also the role-model for the villainous virus in the film *Outbreak*. The film starts as an unidentified illness kills nineteen out of the 26,018 residents of Cedar Creek, a fictitious small north California town, one mile from the Pacific Ocean. Another one hundred are ill with the disease, and no-one knows how many more are infected. Dressed in bio-warfare suits, the army has sealed off the area. Military officials ban any movement of civilians in or out and any that try to make a run for it are blown apart by helicopter gunships. Scientists from the Centers for Disease Control and Prevention track down the virus in a remarkably short time and discover that it looks incredibly like a cartoon version of Ebola. It has a particularly nasty quality in that it can transmit through the air and so everyone in the town is at threat. Being a Hollywood film, a cure is found, removing the need to put an end to the virus by blasting the town off the face of the Earth.

The real Ebola is scary, but in reality slightly less devastating. So far it comes in five varieties, each named after the town or country where it was initially identified – Ebola Zaire, Ebola Sudan, Ebola Reston, Ebola Tai and Ebola Ivory Coast. Ebola itself is the name of the river running through Zaire where the virus first showed its colours. They all look the same down an electron microscope, but they have subtly different characteristics. Ebola Reston, for example, is uniquely nasty because it can transmit from victim to victim through the air. It first came to light in November 1989 in an ape-house just outside Washington DC and probably arrived from the Philippines. The terror of an airborne version of this deadly agent diminished once disease control scientists realised that it could only kill apes. For some unknown reason, while the virus can infect humans, we manage to set up an immune response that chases it away. This generation of the virus was devastating to apes, but benign to humans – looks like we had a lucky escape.

The other four versions of Ebola are less charitable. Ebola Zaire and Ebola Sudan showed up almost simultaneously in 1976. Zaire kills nine out of ten infected people. Sudan kills "only" six out of ten. The disease moves from person to person in the blood and body fluids that spray into the air each time a victim coughs. Avoid contact with blood, faeces, urine, vomit and semen and you should be okay.

The Ebola virus seems to enjoy living in the cells that build small blood vessels. The problem is that, as with most viruses, once the replication cycle is complete the new viruses burst out, destroying the cell. Very soon this tears holes in the blood vessels and they start to leak. If the blood vessels are in the eyes then the whites of the eyes turn a shocking red.

Search as they might, no-one has found where Ebola hides in the wild. A region can be disease-free for years and then it breaks out again. In terms of a global threat to health, the virus doesn't seem to be too important, the reason being that epidemics seem to die out of their own accord, and with stringent hygiene around victims there is no need for the disease to spread once it has been identified. Ebola also has a short period between infection and the appearance of symptoms. This helps health professionals keep the disease under control because they can rapidly identify and isolate all infected individuals.

That is, of course, unless it mutates. The frightening concept is that one form of the virus learns to spread through the air, like Ebola Reston, but carries a warhead that is as devastating as Ebola Zaire. If it then added to its skills the ability to delay disclosure of its presence, and like HIV could spread widely before being detected, that would be the ultimate nightmare – the ultimate superbug.

Marburg has a similar history. It is named after an industrial town in Germany that is not particularly renowned for its possession of weird diseases. It does, however, have ape-houses in a local pharmaceutical factory that produces vaccines. Many vaccines are grown on cells cultured from monkey kidneys and when three men working at Behringwerke AG, the vaccine-producing subsidiary of Hoechst AG, went down with 'flu-like symptoms in August 1967 no-one paid much attention. That was until their eyes turned bright red and their spleens started to swell.

Concern had turned to alarm by September as twenty-three workers lay in agony in Marburg University Hospital. At the same time six other people were spread out in a Frankfurt hospital, all of whom had connections with the German government's Paul Ehrlich Institute. Then, a veterinarian and his wife in Belgrade, Yugoslavia, contracted a similar illness. Fear turned to terror, particularly because two wives were sick. If the disease had come from handling diseased monkeys it would be easy to contain, but with wives of victims now infected this meant that it could also move from person to person – maybe through the air. That's much more difficult to contain.

The symptoms worsened and the victims' glands became swollen and tender. The number of disease-fighting white cells in the victim's blood dropped. Their skin became too sensitive to touch and was covered in rashes. Their throats were so sore that they couldn't eat and needed fluids and nutrition to be fed in via a drip. After ten days they started vomiting, and then their skin started peeling off. In the men, even the skin over their genitals was not spared. The pain was excruciating. Seven died, one man became psychotic and others were left with chronic liver disease.

The uniting feature behind all the primary victims was that they had worked with members from one batch of *Cercopithecus aethiops*, vervet monkeys imported from Uganda via Belgrade. Forty-nine out of the ninety-nine animals in the shipment had also died. The person in Belgrade who had caught the disease was the technician who autopsied the dead monkeys. His wife contracted it while she nursed him.

When a team from the WHO went to Uganda to trace the source of the virus they found it in vervet monkeys and red-tailed monkeys. Blood tests on chimpanzees, baboons, talapoins and gorillas showed signs that they had encountered and fought off the virus. Looking at stored blood samples enabled experts to determine that the disease had been around since at least 1961.

Any hopes that Marburg disease would simply fade into history were dashed after a twenty-year-old Australian tourist spent the summer of 1975 hitchhiking around the southern end of Africa. He died in Johannesburg Hospital, his body riddled with the virus. His girlfriend contracted the disease a couple of days after his death, as did a nurse who had cared for him. Doctors pumped heparin into them to prevent their blood clotting and saved their lives.

A summer 2000 outbreak of Marburg in a gold-mining town in the Democratic Republic of the Congo killed twenty, while seventy died of the disease in an outbreak at the same place the previous year. An Ebola outbreak in Uganda killed 224 people in 2001, and Marburg sprang up in Angola in March 2005, infecting 374 people and killing 329 in a five-month reign of terror. Monitoring this outbreak, the WHO says that the vast majority of cases occurred in Uige Province, where 368 cases and 323 deaths were recorded. These viruses aren't about to lie down quietly.

A Visa to Europe

In northern Nigeria in the Yedseram River valley is Lassa, a village that the rest of the world would never have heard of except for the emergence of a new disease. In the 1950s people in the area started dying horrible deaths, and in 1969 the viral agent was identified. Lassa fever, as it became known, has all the hallmarks of a haemorrhagic fever with patients struck down by massive fevers and coughing up infection-laden dissolved lungs and body contents.

The virus passed simply from person to person by direct contact with blood, secretions in the throat that may get coughed into the air, or urine. The virus gets into semen in large numbers, so sexual intercourse up to three months after recovery from the disease can pass it on. And that is if you do recover – one in eight don't. Unlike Marburg, there is some treatment that can make a little difference. If you identify the disease early enough there is some chance that an antiviral drug called Ribavirin can bring some benefit.

Lassa virus has its main residence in a particular rodent, *Mastomys natalensis*, that thrives in sub-Saharan Africa. Breathing in dust contaminated with dried urine from an infected rodent is enough to strike you down. Some twenty thousand to forty thousand people succumb each year and several thousand die.

While the disease has no reservoir in Europe, the year 2000 saw four Lassa-infected people enter the continent. A twenty-three-year-old female student who had just returned from spending a couple of months in the Ivory Coast and Ghana arrived in Lisbon, Portugal. She was seriously ill and as her condition deteriorated she was flown to the Tropical Medicine Department of Würzburg Hospital, Germany, where she died while being treated on an isolation ward. In March the WHO announced that a 50-year-old British man had returned from a remote rural area in Daru, Sierra Leone, where he was working as a part of the peacekeeping effort. He was seriously ill with Lassa fever and being cared for in the high security isolation unit at Coppetts Wood Hospital in London. April saw a Nigerian national die in Germany where he had been flown by air ambulance for treatment. On July 11, a forty-eight-year-old surgeon developed symptoms of Lassa fever while working in Kenema, Sierra Leone. On July 25, he died in Leiden Hospital, in the Netherlands. Doctors initially thought he had malaria, an easy mistake in the early stages of the illness, and so antiviral treatment wasn't started until it was too late.

In each case, dealing with the initial patient is only the first part of the process as health officials dash around trying to locate anyone who could have been in contact with the person. If the person had made a recent plane journey, the passenger list forms an obvious set of candidates who need to be warned. It's not so easy to locate the people who may have bumped into you in the street or, if hygiene standards are low, could be at risk because they "shared" cutlery and cups in a restaurant.

Home and Away

Haemorrhagic Fever with Renal Syndrome first came to the attention of Western physicians when between 1951 and 1954 some 3,200 of the United Nations forces in Korea got it. It is caused by a hantavirus, an agent that belongs to the bunyavirus family of viruses. The other bunyaviruses (bunyavirus, phlebovirus, nariovirus and tospovirus) have their main home in insects, but hantaviruses live in mice and are transmitted to humans when a person is bitten by infected mites.

In fact, it turns out that there are half a dozen different hantaviruses that cause two different styles of infection. One is the haemorrhagic fever, in which the person's kidneys pack up, and the other is a rapid respiratory failure. This latter form first showed up in the Four Corners region of the United States – New Mexico, Arizona, Colorado and Utah.

The first recorded victim of the respiratory version was twenty-one-year-old Florena Woody, a young Navajo Native American woman who had been living with her twenty-year-old boyfriend, Merrill Bahe, and their five-month-old baby. They lived in a trailer in the tiny reservation town of Littlewater, New Mexico. Merrill was an athlete and both of them were full of life. On April 29, 1993, Florena's shoulders ached so Merrill gave them a gentle rub, but the pain stayed. Four days later she had a high fever and began to cough. On May 6 she visited her doctor to discuss some earlier surgery and mentioned her condition. By May 9 she had deteriorated and was in hospital having difficulty breathing. And then she died. Her lungs had filled with fluid. Five days later, as Merrill drove to her funeral, he too collapsed and died. The lining of his lungs had suddenly become porous and the air spaces become filled with liquid. Their baby survived. Hantavirus had arrived in the United States and was there to stay. CDC reports show that in 1998 thirty people got Hantavirus Pulmonary Syndrome (HPS). They were in twelve different states. Nine cases were fatal.

The frightening thing about this particular virus is that the initial symptoms are indistinguishable from normal 'flu. There is no medical system in the world that has the resources to place every 'flu victim in intensive care, so doctors in areas where the virus exists have to watch carefully and act quickly.

And Bacteria Have Their Own Villains

Viruses aren't the only bio-criminals that make your body fall to pieces. A few types of bacteria are quite keen to get in on the act if they are given the chance.

Rita Ryan woke up one morning with a cough. Nothing unusual and nothing to worry about. Life continued its normal pattern of getting her four-year-old daughter to day care, her six-year-old to school and herself to the college in St Louis, Missouri, where she was teaching general education and business classes. The cough, however, continued. She bought cough mixture in the local pharmacy and presumed that all would be well in a couple of days.

After a week of no improvement she phoned her doctor: "He gave me a prescription for antibiotic medication and over the next two days I started to find some relief," explains Rita. "Then on the third day while I was at work I started to get back pain and felt very bad. That night I woke up in the middle of the night and I had a tremendous pain in the upper middle of my back – the left side of my back. On the morning of March 11, 1999, my husband left home for work and my son went off to school. Then my breathing became very shallow so I called the paramedics. My daughter was with me when the paramedics arrived at the house and she was terrified when they rushed me to the ambulance – she was sure I was dead. She was petrified and, of course, she told my son. They thought that they would never see me again."

St Anthony's Medical Center in St Louis was only five minutes away by ambulance, but by the time Rita arrived at 8:30 am she was slipping into a coma. They didn't expect her to live. "They told my family to prepare for the worst. They didn't think I was going to make it through the night. I had *Streptococcus pneumoniae*. It infected my entire system. I had respiratory failure, renal failure, infected liver, and sepsis (blood poisoning)."

Rita was taken straight to intensive care and put on a respirator to keep her breathing and dialysis to help support her kidneys. She was given massive doses of antibiotics.

For eleven days it was touch and go whether Rita would survive, but slowly her body took on the fight. In the end she lay in a coma for eighteen days while doctors and nurses fought around the clock to save her life. The key thing was to fight the infection and then to get rid of the toxic chemicals from the blood and drain the fluid from the lungs. She also needed eight pints of blood.

"It was twenty days before they let my children come and see me. It was very traumatic for them."

By this time the *S. pneumoniae* had turned Rita's body into a bloody battlefield. Internally her organs were in a desperate state. But the massive scale of the infection became apparent as huge sores started to develop on both of Rita's legs. Rapidly the tissue died and eight-inch by four-inch slabs of skin turned charcoal black – areas the size of a large hand. "It was like frost-bite and went as deep as a third-degree burn," says Rita in a remarkably casual voice. "It all had to be cut away, which left huge open wounds."

Not surprisingly, her body was in shock and all her hair fell out. "I also lost all of my nails and in the end the doctors had to cut off the nail beds from four of my toes."

"My sister-in-law tells me that the nephrologist [kidney specialist] and the respiratory guy were just dedicated to me. There were thirteen staff in all and they were there around the clock. I had nurses that worked double shift – they were continually on the internet trawling for information, and they were doing everything that they could to help me fight this. I had nurses that wouldn't go home at night – and doctors that wouldn't leave my room. They did not want to lose me. I had such a mental constitution that I just wasn't going to give in to this – and I was determined to hold on. My parents slept round the clock in the hospital. My husband was there as much as he could while at the same time looking after the kids. I fought it with every ounce I had – it was the most exhausting fight I have ever had – it took everything out of me. I was thirty-eight when this happened – but I looked as if I was ninety."

On May 4, 1999, after fifty-four days in hospital, Rita went home – the war had been won, though there was still a lot of recovery needed. The total hospital bill was $225,000 – but Rita only had to pay $200, the insurance company picked up the rest. "The medical industry in the US, the physicians and the health insurance, are much maligned. But I have nothing but praise."

"For the next six months I was exhausted – I would take a bath and then have to go and sit down to recuperate for hours. Prior to that I'd never been sick – I've had the normal influenza and things, but nothing serious. At the end of September I managed to get back to work, but I still go back for check-ups every three months. Internally, I am completely healed, but I still have huge scars on my legs."

Rita was lucky. One thousand three hundred people in the US died of group A streptococcal disease in 1998 alone, a further 10,200 had infections that caused a more minor version of the disease. She was also helped by the fact that she didn't smoke or spend time with smokers and she was generally fit. But she still needed antibiotics to tip the balance in her favour. In the near future, recovery from this sort of disease could become more difficult as the CDC also reports that they are finding increasing numbers of this bug that are resistant to one or more antibiotics.

CHAPTER 10 –
THE VIRAL GOOD GUYS

Great fleas have little fleas upon their backs to bite 'em,
And little fleas have lesser fleas, and so ad infinitum.
And the great fleas themselves, in turn, have greater fleas to go on;
While these again have greater still, and greater still, and so on.[1]

Do fleas have fleas on them? Well, maybe not, but bacteria have viruses to contend with. Yes, bacteria can be infected and killed by viruses. So, before we completely write off viruses as the no-hope bad-guy, the ultimate villains who have no hope of reform, and say that all viruses should be locked away permanently with no hope of parole, we need to have a brief look at bacteriophages – phages for short. They may not have a high profile at the moment, but there is every possibility that our children will talk of these with much the same sense of familiarity that we refer to antibiotics – and for similarly perceived miraculous powers. It may even be that the miracle title for phages is more justified and longer-lived than it has been for antibiotics. In the face of apparently untreatable bacterial disease, these microbes-with-a-mission may prove to be our knights in shining armour.

In Tbilisi, deep in the heart of the Caucasus Mountains, is the central hospital of the republic of Georgia. Like all hospitals, it has its fair share of multi-drug resistant bacteria. Unlike most, though, the members of staff are not overly concerned about this issue, and this almost relaxed attitude is not caused by negligence or complacency. They have phages.

The first person to realise that phages exist was E. H. Hankin from the Pasteur Institute in Paris, who in 1896 reported that water from the Ganges and Jumma rivers in India killed some bacteria.[2] He was particularly struck by the fact that something in the water could kill *Vibrio Cholerae*, the bug that causes cholera, and suggested that whatever the agent was, it was capable of restricting or reducing the number of outbreaks of this potentially lethal disease. Hankin never found out what was causing this, but he did discover that it could pass through porcelain filters and be made ineffective by heating.

English bacteriologist Edward Twort was the next person to move the phage story forward, when in 1915 he found that he could isolate from sewage an unknown substance that would leave dead patches in smooth lawns of bacteria growing on culture plates – biological bullet-holes. Twort did not pursue this finding, but we now know that phages exist wherever you find bacteria – just one millilitre of seawater can contain a million phages.

Two years later, French-Candian Félix H. d'Hérelle made a similar discovery. Bizarrely, the subject of his investigation was locust diarrhoea in Mexico. During an invasion of insects, local Indians showed d'Hérelle a place where the ground was strewn with dead and dying locusts. Clearly they had a blackish diarrhoea. Félix H. d'Hérelle found that sick insects could infect healthy ones, and that spreading the diarrhoea on leaves and feeding these to healthy insects was equally effective in passing on the infection.

He started to culture the bacteria that he suspected were growing in the locust excrement. It was when he looked at culture plates where he had smeared some of the muck that he paused for thought. Bacteria grew across the plate, *Coccobacilli*. That much he had expected. But clear spots appeared in the bacterial lawn. Something was munching the *Coccobacilli*. "In a flash I had understood," said d'Hérelle. "What caused my clear spots was in fact an invisible microbe… a virus parasitic to bacteria."[3]

Back in the Pasteur Institute in Paris, d'Hérelle repeated this experiment using excrement not from locusts, but a Paris-based squadron that was struck down with dysentery. Again the same finding. Nature, declared d'Hérelle, had provided humankind with a living, natural weapon against germs.

One misconception that he had was that there was only one type of phage and that some bacteria develop a resistance to it. In reality, there are many phages, each targeted at a specific population of bacteria and bacteria have limited defensive strategies. Sadly, though, this error in understanding was to set back the cause by possibly half a century or more.

Space Vehicles on Earth

With the advent of electron microscopes we can now see these little critters, and strange they look too. They are around one-fortieth the size of the average bacterium and bear a remarkable resemblance to Apollo's lunar module, which first settled down on the Moon's surface in 1969. A large polyhedron sits on the top of a short stalk, and at the bottom of the stalk are six spindly legs. Phages can only infect bacteria – a fact that makes them extremely interesting for anyone trying to kill disease. They do so by landing on the surface of the bug and locking the ends of their legs to specific cell surface receptors. These receptors are highly indicative of the type of bacterium that the phage has encountered, and explains its specificity. The next stage is to compact their stalk. This drives a hypodermic needle-like tube through the bacterial wall and DNA contained in the polyhedral head passes into the bacterium.

Like all viruses, this genetic material sets to work generating new copies of the phages, often up to two hundred in half an hour. When they burst out they destroy the bacterial cell, resulting in one dead bacterium and loads of new phages looking for more victims. Were each of the two hundred phages to infect new bacteria you could theoretically have forty thousand phages within an hour, and repeating this twice more would give 1.6 billion within two hours of the initial encounter.

It is an impressive scale-up that is potentially wonderful – a self-propagating and highly selective therapeutic agent. In theory, you need only give a diseased person a few phage particles – the infecting bacteria will generate the rest. Better than that, as soon as all the bacteria are dead there is nowhere for the phages to go, so they too die out. It's a self-limiting infection.

So why don't we buy phages off the shelf whenever we are ill? The problem is that phages have proved extremely difficult to handle and use and we now know that you have to match your phage exactly to your offending bacterium. Many bacteria didn't respond, giving the illusion of resistance when in fact the scientists were simply using the wrong type of phage. Manufacturing processes also involved growing phages on batches of bacteria. In earlier chapters we saw how the death of bacteria could cause fever, as all their contents spilt into the person's blood-stream. In a similar way, busted bacteria from the culture media could cause violent reactions if injected along with phages. The complex separation was not possible in early trials, although the technology needed has come along fairly recently.

Eli Lilly did start to manufacture therapeutic phages in the United States in the 1930s, but this operation was completely eclipsed by the post-war antibiotic explosion. Suddenly there was no need to make a pact with nature and employ one bug against another. Instead, companies could mass-produce chemicals, pack them in pills and we could pop them in our mouths whenever we became unwell. Everyone knew how wonderful antibiotics were. Marketing was simple. Who needs phages?

With antibiotics on the run, the answer could well be "we all do". So we return to Tbilisi. Félix H. d'Hérelle's work came to the attention of none other than Stalin's government. This must have been thrilling for d'Hérelle as, despite his aristocratic upbringing, he was a passionate Communist and ended up dedicating a book he had written to Stalin. In 1934 he accepted an invitation from Sergo Ordjonikidze, the People's Commissar of Heavy Industry, to help them set up a research institute that would exploit these minute miracles. The KGB appeared to have been suspicious of anything that came from the West, but the Eliava Institute was set up on the banks of the river Mtkvary at the Institute of Bacteriology in Tbilisi. D'Hérelle sent supplies, equipment and books, most of which he paid for himself, and in 1934 he and his wife travelled to the Institute to work there for six months. He declined the offer of a full-time post.

This activity was set against Western medical science's mood of disbelief about phages. A 1931 review commissioned by the American Medical Association's Council of Pharmacy and Chemistry studied one hundred and fifty scientific references and concluded that "experimental studies of the lytic [bacteria-bursting] agent called 'bacteriophage' have not disclosed its nature. D'Hérelle's theory that the material is a living parasite of bacteria has not been proved. On the contrary, the facts appear to indicate that the material is inanimate, possibly an enzyme."[4] Let's not be too hard on the reviewers. In the 1930s scientists had only a scant knowledge of viruses, and in many ways their analysis was remarkably good. Phages are not living organisms, they are viruses. The report's authors were unconvinced about the value of phages, if they exist at all, but did concede that "[only] in the treatment of local staphylococcic infections and perhaps cystitis has evidence at all convincing been presented."

In Tbilisi things could not have been more different and one of the Eliava Institute's first successes was a powerful dysentery phage used by the Red Army during the Second World War. Many other triumphs were reported against diseases including typhoid, parathyroid fevers, cholera, pus-producing infections and urinary diseases. The Institute prepared phages in solutions that could be injected into the skin, muscle, directly into veins, into the space around the intestines or into the gut itself. Some injections went into the heart, lungs and arteries that feed the brain.

As well as being a potential therapeutic agent, one early use of phages was in helping bacteriologists identify bacteria. With an individual phage infecting only an individual strain of bacteria, you could test a bacterial culture by exposing it to a phage library, a carefully catalogued collection of phages. Only one phage would affect the culture and then you would have identified your bug. Scientists at the Eliava built up a library of hundreds of phages to enable this phage-typing.

For two reasons it is a shame that this work happened in the Soviet Union. First, the West was deeply sceptical of any claim that emanated from the USSR and so ignored any statements of success. More tragically, since the collapse of the republic, funding to this area of science has virtually dried up and the infrastructure that a scientific community requires has crumbled. Phages need to be kept in a refrigerator, but with frequent and prolonged power-cuts, the refrigerators fail and the phages fall to pieces. Phage therapy used to be a standard feature of pre-glasnost Georgia, with twelve hundred people employed to produce tons of tablets, liquid preparations and sprays of carefully selected mixtures of phages – some were even packaged in enemas. Some were used in treatment, others to prevent disease, and they were shipped everywhere across the Soviet Union. You could buy them over the counter, or get them from your doctor.

Under the orders of the Soviet Ministry of Health, hundreds of thousands of samples of pathogenic bacteria were sent to the Institute from all over the Union, most of which revealed some form of phage. In fact, trawling sewage is a very good way of finding them. The scale of work was impressive. Between 1983 and 1985 they studied the growth, biochemical features and phage sensitivity of 2,038 strains of *Staphylococcus*, 1,128 of *Streptococcus*, 328 of *Proteus*, 373 of *Pseudomonas aeruginosa* and 622 of *Clostridium*. Excitingly, some phages were found that had a moderately broad range of action.

Once again disease thrives on conflict, and the fighting in near-by Abkhasia left 350,000 refugees in a country of five million people and cut off major transport and power lines. Georgia has no money for science. But the drawing back of the Iron Curtain has been accompanied by a renewed interest in the East. With the potential of investment from the West it is now, however, the East's turn to be sceptical of foreign intentions. Given the potential for solving the looming crisis of antibiotic resistance it is a shame that progress has been so slow.

In Britain, Willie Smith and Michael Huggins at the Institute for Animal Health, Huntingdon, carried out a series of studies looking for phage that could tackle diarrhoea in calves. Their source material was sewage from treatment plants, from cattle markets and from slurry pits, "the idea being that you would most likely find these phages in areas where you got a collection of shit."[5] They injected *E. coli* bacteria into mice and the mice died. They injected the same dose of bacteria into other mice along with a shot of phages and the mice lived. The phages were more effective than numerous antibiotics – tetracycline, streptomycin, ampicillin or trimethoprim/sulfafurazole. In calves they found that phages give a very high level of protection. Phages could protect animals from diarrhoea or cure them when they had it.

Skin grafts placed on people who have suffered burns are notoriously prone to loss through infection. The prime culprit is the bacterium *Pseudomonas aeruginosa*. Working with animals, James Soothill from the University of Birmingham found that suitably targeted phages could wipe out the bacterial infection and prevent this occurring.[6]

After a slow start momentum is gathering. In 1993 Dr Richard Carlton formed Exponential Biotherapies, based in Rockville, Maryland. This was the first American company devoted exclusively to phage therapy work. Five years later, Intralytix, another company determined to bring phage therapy to the medical market, started in Baltimore.

Canadian venture capitalist Caisey Harlingten took an interest in phages after reading an article about them in *Scientific American* and set up Phage Therapeutics International. Based in Seattle, this company made the news on September 16, 1999, when they treated a woman in Toronto who had contracted a potentially fatal bacterial infection during heart surgery. The bacteria had moved into her heart. They appeared to be resistant to all known antibiotics – it was an MRSA and her outcome looked grim. At this point her family appealed to Phage International Inc. and got permission from the company, their doctors and the hospital to use a phage they had found which targets *S. aureus*. Doctors sprayed the phage directly into the artery that fed the woman's heart and nearly twenty-four hours later pretty well all traces of the bacteria had been wiped out. Phages saved the day, but not her life. Sadly, the woman died two months later, but her doctors pointed out that this was due to the heart condition, not the bacterial infection.

Engineering Resistance

Now here's a turn up for the books. One of the factors that could limit the usefulness of phages is that they are viruses. We've spent a long time getting worried about viruses' ability to cause havoc, but while some viruses do beat the system, our bodies are quite good at hunting them down and sweeping them away if they are free-floating in blood. To make up for this, patients therefore need three or four doses of phages. But what if you could engineer a phage that can evade the body's housekeeping system? It is exactly what some scientists have managed to do.

Carl Merril and colleagues at the Laboratory of Biochemical Genetics, at the National Institutes of Health, Washington, DC, have injected wild-type phages into mice and then collected any phages that remained in the animals seven hours later. To have survived, they must have side-stepped the eviction process. These were grown in culture and injected into a second set of mice. Repeating this nine times they selected phages that had strong survival instincts. The results were impressive. Survival after eighteen hours was sixteen thousand times higher in the new strain of phages when compared to the wild-type particles.[7]

Bacteria, however, may have one more trick up their sleeve. Research at Michigan State University in East Lansing indicates that they can commit suicide. This may not at first seem to be a particularly strong move, but Larry Snyder and colleagues have seen bacteria do this after they are infected with phage. As far as the individual bacterium is concerned, suicide is obviously the end of the line, but this selfless act means that the phage can't multiply. The rest of the colony is spared. So maybe after mass use, bacteria will develop a novel version of resistance.

The West could also continue to learn much from former eastern-bloc countries. Stefan Slopek and colleagues in Wroclaw, Poland, have now treated infections in 550 people with various phages and obtained positive results in 508 cases – that's nine out of ten. Not bad, particularly when 518 of these patients had infections that were resistant to antibiotics. It is easy to criticise the trials because they do not have classic "control arms" that enable a treatment group to be compared with a group of people who receive no treatment. Still, the impressive results speak for themselves.[8]

Sometimes literature is more perceptive than science, as is the case with Nobel Prize winner Sinclair Lewis's book *Arrowsmith*. The plot tells of Martin Arrowsmith, a rather ordinary fellow who gets his first taste of medicine as a 14-year-old and ends up travelling around the world using phages to treat his patients. Lewis depicts Arrowsmith as a person caught between his idealism and commercialism. Intriguingly, the book won Lewis a Pulitzer Prize, which he declined because he felt that Pulitzers were meant to be awarded for books that celebrate American wholesomeness, and his novels were critical of it. However, in finding material for his plot he could inadvertently have chosen the technology that has most hope of leading us into a healthier future with bacteria once again on the run.

Only time will tell whether phages will enter our popular medical vocabulary. Many scientists in the West are still sceptical, but the evidence from the East seems strong.

CHAPTER 11 –
PR IS FOR PRIONS

Bacteria are nasty because they are microscopic self-contained units that can live alongside or within an animal or human being and cause trouble. Viruses create mayhem because they bury themselves into your cells and carry out a *coup d'état*, reorganising the cell's activity to serve its purposes. But what of an infective agent that is already part of yourself? What of prions?

Let me offer a few basic points of dogma. One: an infectious disease needs a pathogen. There are diseases that, as far as we know, have no agent involved, like gallstones and skin cancer. Consequently there is no way that you can catch these from another person, or for that matter from another animal. They might be diseases, but by definition they are not infectious. Two: the pathogen must be able to reproduce new copies of itself. If you need one thousand bacteria to cause a disease, and those bacteria moved in but couldn't increase their numbers, two things would happen. First the disease would not take hold, and secondly it couldn't pass on to anybody else. Again, as an infective disease, it would fail. Three: to reproduce, a pathogen needs to contain all the information needed to build new copies of itself; it needs a genetic memory bank. Bacteria and viruses both contain either DNA or RNA – gene-bearing genetic material. This gives them all the instructions needed to build new copies of the infective agent. Ever since Francis Crick and James Watson discovered the structure of DNA in the 1960s, every biologist has accepted that this is the way, the only way, that biology stores and transmits information.

It makes sense, but like most, this three-part dogma is flawed. Prions have become the ugly fact that destroys a beautiful theory. They are infectious lumps of protein that carry their devastation from animal to animal, replicating upon arrival, but possessing no genetic information. "Fifteen years ago," comments Stanley Prusiner, the discoverer of prions, "I evoked a good deal of scepticism when I proposed that the infectious agents causing certain degenerative disorders of the central nervous system in animals and, more rarely, in humans might consist of protein and nothing else. At the time, the notion was heretical."[1]

Prusiner added insult to injury by going on to suggest that such a putative infectious agent could operate by converting normal protein molecules into dangerous ones simply by inducing the benign molecules to change their shape. To most scientists who knew anything about diseases, the whole idea was preposterous.

The fog now appears to be clearing. Prusiner and other scientists have shown that prion proteins are the unifying factor behind a series of previously mysterious neurodegenerative diseases, often referred to as spongiform encephalopathies. The name derives from the holes that develop in the brains of people affected by these conditions − holes that give the brain the appearance of bath sponges. Scrapie in sheep and goats is the most common form of the disease. Animals slowly lose co-ordination and have subtle changes in temperament. They often start to rub themselves against fixed objects, scraping off their wool − hence the disease's name. Weight loss despite a good appetite, biting themselves and hopping like a rabbit are also common signs. A sudden noise can cause an animal to have a fit and fall down. European sheep first showed signs of it in the mid-1700s and the first US case was in 1947 in a Michigan flock that had been imported from Britain via Canada. It has now been found in over 950 flocks in the US. Australia and New Zealand are the only countries that claim to be free of the disease.

Mink, elk, mule deer, cats and cows all have their own versions of the disease, and human beings are not exempt. Kuru is a disease known only among the Fore people of Papua New Guinea. This tribe took the unusual step of honouring the dead by eating them, and treated their brains as something of a delicacy. People with "laughing death", as the Fore people called it, died after they lost their co-ordination and became demented. At first people would become unsteady as they walked around. They would slowly lose control of their eyes, hands and voices. As the disease progressed they became incapable of walking without support and their muscles had shock-like jerks. They would burst out laughing and then be depressed. Toward the end of their lives sufferers would be incapable of sitting up and would have little control over their muscles. They'd be incontinent and have difficulty swallowing. It was an awful way to die.[2]

Over a twenty-year period between the 1950s and late 1960s, over three thousand of the thirty-five thousand Fore people died from the disease.[3] Eight times more women than men contracted the disease, which isn't surprising now that we know the cause, because women were the chief players in the mortuary cannibalism. Children were also highly susceptible, but again this makes sense because they joined the women in their cannibalistic work. To make matters worse, kuru victims were highly regarded as sources of food, because the layer of fat on victims who died quickly resembled pork.

Initially the people who went to Papua New Guinea to investigate kuru thought that it must be genetic; after all, it was confined to this inbred population. Once this theory was discounted, they moved on to look for a "slow virus".

In 1965 D. Carlton Gajdusek, from the National Institutes of Health, Bethesda, Maryland, performed a vital experiment. He took brain tissue from people who had died of kuru and injected it into chimpanzees. Within eighteen to thirty-six months, all the chimpanzees developed an identical range of symptoms. The disease was certainly infectious, but the period between inoculation and symptoms was far greater than anything seen before. It called for a new type of infective agent. Intriguingly, before Prusiner's 1982 publication in *Science* had set prions firmly on the map, Gajdusek had taken part-share of the 1976 Nobel Prize in Physiology or Medicine for identifying that kuru was a totally new form of infectious agent that had similarities to the recently identified hepatitis virus. His best guess was that the unidentified agent was a "slow virus".

Prusiner tells how his interest in prion diseases started in 1972 when he was a neurology resident at the University of California, San Francisco, and a patient he was caring for died of CJD. He was shocked by this disease, which in two months destroyed the woman's brain while leaving the rest of her body physically unaffected. There were none of the classic signs of infection – no sign of a fever, no immune response in her blood, no sign of disease-combating cells in the fluid bathing her brain. Prusiner was simply told that she had a "slow virus". "Next, I learned that scientists were unsure if a virus was really the cause of CJD since the causative infectious agent had some unusual properties," says Prusiner in an autobiography written for the Nobel Foundation.[4] "The amazing properties of the presumed causative 'slow virus' captivated my imagination and I began to think that defining the molecular structure of this elusive agent might be a wonderful research project. The more that I read about CJD and the seemingly related diseases – kuru of the Fore people of New Guinea and scrapie of sheep – the more captivated I became."

When Prusiner set up a small research laboratory in 1974 with the hope of tracking down the causative agent, he was expecting to find a small virus. Many people warned him that this was a hopeless area of research. But he persisted. He was intrigued by work carries out by Tikvah Alper and her colleagues at Hammersmith Hospital, London, who by 1972 had isolated an agent that caused scrapie in sheep and found that it was highly resistant to anything that could damage DNA.[5]

The more research he did, the more puzzled he became, because like Alper's work, time and again the results indicated that neither DNA nor RNA was present. Infected brain material still passed on the disease even after it had been exposed to ultra-violet light or alkylating chemicals, both of which destroy DNA. But infectivity requires genetics – everyone knows that – and genetics demands DNA or RNA. He also found that scrapie infectivity was reduced by any procedure that specifically damaged protein. Maybe, just maybe, the agent was just a protein. By 1982 he had purified an agent that was "proteinaceous" and "infective" and named it a prion[6] – presumably he thought that this sounded better than proin, which would have been a more natural derivative!

Remarkably, this prion was a single protein and because scientists love abbreviating everything it is normally called PrP (Prion Protein).

It is amusing to look back on Gajdusek's Nobel Prize. The award was given although everyone was aware that he hadn't identified the agent. Hence his suggestion of a "slow virus". The Nobel committee acknowledged that the mystery was finally solved when they awarded Prusiner the 1997 prize for Medicine or Physiology for his discovery of prions.

Thankfully, kuru has all but died out since the cannibalism practice ceased in 1959. No children born after that year have suffered the disease. Sadly the world's interest in prion diseases didn't die out with the demise of kuru, because another crisis loomed in the form of bovine spongiform encephalitis, better known as "mad cow disease", and its human spin-off of "new variant-CJD", both of which have a uniting feature – prions.

The World of the Prion

So what do we know about prions? The 1980s produced the discovery that every mammal investigated has genes that enable it to build prion proteins – including mice, hamsters and humans. This led to a dilemma. If all mammals made them, why did only some get sick? Maybe prions had nothing to do with disease, or maybe there were two different forms of the protein.

We now know that in human cells the gene for prion protein is part of chromosome 20. No-one knows what the protein does, but it exists in nerve cells in the brain. Like all proteins, it is built from a chain of amino acids that folds and spirals into specific shapes. The shape is determined by the sequence of the amino acids.

In healthy people the prion protein molecule is packed with corkscrewing a-helices, which are distinct features of many proteins. In people with CJD the helical structure is replaced with flat sheets. The unusual feature is that both conformations of the protein can have identical sequences of amino acids. The infective nature of kuru came about because when people ate brains containing altered prion protein, this novel protein seems to have formed a template in their cells causing their naturally occurring and healthy prion protein to change shape. Quite what this altered version does is again a mystery, but it is clearly not good for the brain.

This explains how prion diseases can be caught, but it doesn't explain how they occur spontaneously and how they can be inherited by standard methods of genetic inheritance. The clue to this conundrum came from a German man who was dying of Gerstmann-Straussler-Scheinker disease, an illness that looked very much like CJD and had afflicted his family. When Prusiner studied the prion protein's gene in his cells they found that it differed in one place – just one difference out of seven hundred and fifty letters of code. This alteration was enough to cause the whole molecule to form in a different way. Instead of the healthy helices, there were the disease-forming sheets. Since then, around twenty families have been found around the world who have single letter changes in the prion gene that leave them susceptible to this form of dementia.

CJD affects people worldwide, striking one in a million people, typically at around the age of sixty. The majority of cases appear to be spontaneous outbreaks of the disease, but some fifteen per cent have a genetic link to other family members and a small number result from the infective agent being introduced inadvertently during medical treatment.

The fact that prion protein is a very normal part of the body explains why it was so difficult to track down. Being part of "self", prions will never be spotted by the immune system, so they will never be detected as "foreign", and there will never be an immune response to the disease.

From BSE to nvCJD

In November 1986 a disturbing disease started to show up in UK cattle. Vets notified the Central Veterinary Laboratory in Weybridge about two cows from herds in different parts of England. They had abnormal neurological symptoms. Farmers were used to sheep having scrapie, but now beef cattle and dairy cows seemed to have a similar condition. The disease acquired the popular name of "Mad Cow Disease", but was more officially called bovine spongiform encephalitis, or BSE. The assumption was that they must have caught the disease by eating cattle feed enriched with meat and bone meal generated by grinding up the bits of sheep that butchers don't sell over the counter. These bits include brain and spinal nerves – material rich in prions.

In 1988, the UK government's Ministry of Agriculture, Fisheries and Food took the issue seriously and in July banned any mammalian protein going into ruminant feed and prohibited the use of mammalian meat and bone-meal in any farm livestock feed. Sadly this was not taken with the full degree of urgency, and contaminated feed remained on some farms for many years. At the same time the government started a planned system of culling animals with the disease. The busiest year was 1992, when 43,154 cattle were slaughtered.

The epidemic reached its peak in 1993, since when the number of cases has fallen. By the end of 1995 a total of 186,193 cattle had been slaughtered and the epidemic was in sharp decline. The number of confirmed cases of the disease had dropped by forty per cent compared to the previous year and the following year saw them halve again. Farmers were beginning to relax, feeling that at last the worst was over and their firm measures were enabling them to move toward the goal of BSE-free herds. It would take time but the best advice seemed to be saying that everything was under control.

It had been hard for UK herds, but no-one other than farmers was too concerned. In any case, the government paid the farmers good compensation for every animal killed. Scrapie had been around for hundreds of years and there was no indication that it had ever crossed the species barrier and entered humans, so if this was just a new form of scrapie, and it was already well on its way to virtual eradication, why worry?

Then the bombshell. I was in Paris in the spring of 1996 on a few days' holiday, just before the birth of my first son, when my wife and I started seeing news placards indicating that all was not well with UK beef. A paper published in the medical journal The Lancet by the UK's National CJD Surveillance Unit in Edinburgh announced the Unit's shocking conclusion: "These cases [of human brain disease] appear to represent a new variant of CJD (nvCJD), which may be unique to the UK. This raises the possibility that they are causally linked to BSE."[7] There were other possibilities, but the most likely was that scrapie had given rise to BSE and BSE to a new human brain disease – nvCJD.[8]

The 1996 announcement sent waves of panic sweeping across the meat-eating populations of Europe and North America, the UK's main markets for beef. The question on everyone's lips was "Is beef safe?". The uncertainty in any answers was followed by extreme changes in the beef market. Exports of beef and any bovine product from the UK were instantly banned as country after country threw up trade barriers. A market that had been worth £500 million a year vanished. UK public confidence in eating beef, or for that matter any meat products, plummeted and domestic sales fell initially by almost a third and some commentators were surprised it didn't drop further. Sales of processed beef products have suffered even more with beefburgers falling forty-three per cent, beef sausages forty-nine per cent and pork and beef sausages down forty-six per cent. UK agriculture was plunged into crisis.

It's true that even before the BSE crisis there was a downward trend in the UK market for frozen red meat products such as beefburgers and grills. Sales of these products dropped from eighty-five thousand tonnes in 1980 to just over sixty-five thousand tonnes in 1995. But in 1996, hit by BSE, the market fell to forty-five thousand tonnes, losing as much in a few months as it had in the previous fifteen years. Across the European Union consumers were nervous and beef's share of the meat market fell from twenty-four per cent in 1995 to an estimated twenty-one per cent in 1996. It might not seem much, but the bottom line is that EU beef consumption fell by one million tonnes in 1996.

Another raft of protective measures were established by European Union bosses, written down in the Florence Framework and unleashed on UK agriculture. All cattle over thirty months old were to be slaughtered and removed from the human food chain. This ensured that no cattle old enough to have been fed meat and bone-meal could stay in the herd and land up on a butcher's slab. Secondly, feeding mammalian meat and bone meal to any farm animal was banned. Thirdly, any part of an animal that was liable to harbour prions, for example the brain and spinal cord, had to be removed at the slaughterhouse and destroyed. Finally, a new set of regulations came into force to oversee the running of slaughterhouses, rendering plants, feed mills and farms. Every animal in the UK's herd now has its own passport and identity number enabling its every movement to be traced by the computerised Cattle Tracing Scheme. This alone cost

£36 million to set up and run for a year, and the government agreed to pick up the bill.

On June 10, 1996, the Government launched a feed recall scheme to ensure that all contaminated feed was removed from farms – this was completed by the end of July. On December 16 of the same year the UK government introduced a selective cull procedure that aimed to remove suspect cattle from the UK herd.

By autumn 2001, 5.1 million cattle had been slaughtered under the "Over Thirty Month" scheme, and a further 77,343 had been culled because they had lived alongside cattle that developed symptoms of the disease. An additional 10,971 have been killed because they were offspring of known BSE infected cattle.

Another question that people wanted to ask was "How many people would suffer the disease?". This one has been more difficult to answer and five years later epidemiologists are still unable to say what the scale of the epidemic could be. There are two problems. First, no available test can reliably say whether someone who is living has CJD. All you can do is wait for symptoms to show up. There is consequently no way of knowing the size of the pool of infection. It may be tens, hundreds, thousands – we just don't know. Secondly, assuming that nvCJD behaves in a similar manner to kuru, the incubation time for the disease will be anything from three years to thirty. This means that we won't know until somewhere around 2010 what the real state of the situation is likely to be.

By June 2000 there had been seventy-four cases of probable or confirmed nvCJD in the UK, sixty-three of whom had died. But still no-one could say whether the epidemic was over or just starting and some evidence suggested that the number of affected people could increase. In 1995, when the disease first emerged, there were three deaths. In both 1996 and 1997 there were ten victims and in 1998 the figure rose to eighteen.[9]

A cluster of cases around the small Leicestershire village of Queniborough re-ignited fears. Glen Day, thirty-five, and Pamela Beyless, twenty-four, died in October 1998 and 19-year-old Stacey Robinson had died two months earlier. Then in May 2000 a nineteen-year-old man died at Leicester Royal Infirmary and all the indications were that he had succumbed to nvCJD. On top of this a fifth local twenty-four-year-old person had symptoms of the disease. Is this significant? Is it a quirk of statistics? The year 2000 went on to record twenty-eight cases of people dying. Epidemiologists held their breaths. Would this growth continue? Was the epidemic just starting? A research letter published in *The Lancet* stated that the number of people with symptoms of nvCJD had increased by twenty-three per cent each year since 1994 and that death from the disease had increased by one third each year since 1995.[10]

There was, however, a possible glimmer of light. Azra Ghani and colleagues at the Wellcome Trust Centre for the Epidemiology of Infectious Disease at the University of Oxford, UK, calculated that the maximum number of people affected by nvCJD will be one hundred and thirty-six thousand. This still looks like a lot of people, but it is many less than the millions feared by the European Union Scientific Steering Committee.[11] They also stress that this is the maximum number – the real figure could be considerably lower.

Indeed 2000 turned out to the be the worst year of the epidemic, and each year since numbers have dropped off to the point that there were only nine deaths in 2004 and two in 2005. For those affected this is devastating, but the source of mass panic appears to be receding.

Epidemiological Forensics

While the news media sit around waiting to count coffins, epidemiologists, biological scientists and policy makers are scratching their heads looking for the trail of evidence that should show why this outbreak occurred. It would be interesting to know, but more importantly, it might prevent a repeat. For example, if feeding of meat and bone-meal is a serious risk to the health of cattle and humans, then other countries, including the US, need to follow the UK's lead and outlaw the practice.

Prion disease seems to have gained this new entry into humans as a two step process. The scrapie-causing protein in sheep, scPrP, was capable of re-modelling the bovine PrP so that BSE broke out. This bovinePrP was then able to change the shape of the prion protein in humans, a feat that had not been accomplished by scPrP.

If that was the route, then why hasn't this happened earlier? The most probable answer points the finger of blame at changes in the way that carcasses were rendered to reclaim bits of protein. In the late 1970s the hydrocarbon solvent extraction method used in rendering offal from sheep, cattle, pigs and chickens began to be abandoned. This left the meat and bone-meal with a higher fat content and so it was a more valuable commodity. Unfortunately, it appears that this solvent was also inadvertently smashing up the prion protein, thus preventing it from being passed from one generation of animal to the next.

John Collinge from the Medical Research Council Prion Unit at Imperial College in London, is not sure. He believes that cannibalism is the cause. Just as feeding humans to humans leads to kuru, feeding cattle to cattle leads to BSE. Further, he believes that the epidemic's timing had little to do with the changes in the rendering process and more to do with the number of infectious cases reaching a critical threshold. In August 2000 his research group caused another stir when they suggested that there was a possibility that BSE could also hide in chickens, sheep and pigs.

Prusiner and his Scottish colleague Mike Scott have produced another possible theory. They think that sheep may have been able to induce BSE because they produce two variants of prions. The assumption has been that sheep have their normal prion and the scPrP, but in the summer of 2000 these researchers released data suggesting that sheep can "produce more than one type of prion. One was the scrapie prion which killed them – but we believe at least some were also making the BSE prion."[12] Prusiner says that he has now stopped eating sheep meat.

There are also fears that CJD in all its forms can be passed from human to human via surgical instruments. In 1977 a sixty-nine-year-old woman had a steel electrode inserted into her brain. She was being treated for epilepsy. After the treatment the electrode was rigorously sterilised by exposing it to a combination of benzene, ethanol and formaldehyde vapour for forty-eight hours. It was later used to treat a twenty-three-year-old woman and a 17-year-old man.

All three died of CJD and the most likely explanation is that the 69-year-old woman had the disease first, and the needle had carried altered prion proteins into the other two brains. Charles Weissmann and colleagues at the MRC Prion Unit at Imperial College set up an experiment aimed at simulating this situation using scrapie-infected sheep brain and specially engineered mice. They found that not only could prions survive through the sterilisation procedure, they were more potent than prions that were inoculated straight from one brain to another. Furthermore, they found that an instrument only needed to be in contact with infected material for five minutes before it became loaded with prions.

Collinge believes that this raises the possibility that steel surgical instruments could be a perpetual source of infection. It is particularly nasty because there is no way of identifying carriers of the disease, so there is no way of isolating instruments that have been used on high-risk people and the cost of throwing away surgical tools after each use would be impossible to bear.

Ripples in a Pond

The lesson from the UK is that turning a blind eye to a problem and hoping that it will go away is no way to tackle a disease crisis. It is a shame then that other countries haven't taken more seriously the possibility that their livestock could be affected. Many countries were quick to claim that their herds were clear, when in reality no one was doing any testing. But slowly that started to change. At a time when the UK had the source of its infection under control, other countries started to wake up to the threat. In many ways you can argue that UK beef is now the safest in the world – it is certainly the most monitored and scrutinised.

Between 1986 and 2001, although ninety-eight per cent of BSE cases worldwide were in the UK, two per cent occurred elsewhere. By 2001 a total of eighteen European countries recorded one or more case. Between 2001 and 2003 Canada, Israel and Japan announced that they too had cattle that were affected. With action having had a positive impact in the UK and surveillance increasing elsewhere, it is not surprising that by 2003 some 55 per cent of all BSE cases were now outside the UK. This was also the year that the USA discovered its first case of BSE, and in July 2004 it implemented a new programme of testing among high-risk cattle.[13] This picked up one infected animal in 2005, and suggested that the level of infection wasn't huge. But it also showed that the USA's herd wasn't completely free of the disease, and points to a need for care and vigilance if they are not going to play with fire.

And Then Confusion

Just as everyone seemed to have got bored with BSE two more crises came along to trouble scientists and politicians alike. The public need to be worried as well. The first stemmed from a report in the well-respected *British Medical Journal*[13] casting doubt over the theory that new variant CJD came from eating infected cattle at all. The report's author, a Scottish public health expert named George Venter, claims that the disease was naturally occurring and always present, but that the apparent increase in the numbers of cases is due to increased observation – if you look more thoroughly for something you stand a good chance of finding more of it. If he is right the entire culling episode was a fiasco.

Not surprisingly, his theory has met with criticism from those who would look very silly if it was ever proved to be correct.

Then came another bombshell. The UK government had a longstanding concern that BSE may have been present in the nation's sheep flock. If this proved to be the case then the culling programme would have to be extended to wipe out millions of sheep as well. Before performing this drastic course of action, government scientists embarked on a quarter of a million pound research project to look for any traces of BSE in the brains of sheep.

The only way to do this was to feed animal brains to mice that have been bred so that they are particularly susceptible to the disease. If BSE-causing prions are present these mice will develop symptoms and die. As the trial was nearing its end, the news appeared to be bad. Mice were dying. It looked as if sheep were an endangered species in the British Isles.

But the next twist in this odd tale was one of the most bizarre. It turns out that for the past few years, government scientists had been mixing up their samples. They had been feeding minced-up cow brains to the mice instead of brain material from sheep. Everyone knew that there was BSE in cow brains so no wonder the mice became ill. The announcement of this farce was made by sending faxes late one Wednesday night, with all the appearance that the officials concerned hoped that no-one would spot them.

The bottom line is that more than two decades after the first reported case of new variant CJD we are still unsure of its origins and don't know for certain how far the causative prions have spread through our food chain.

Whatever the long-term scale and outcome of the UK's prion disease epidemic, or its occurrence in any other part of the world, one lesson has been learned – never underestimate the ability of infectious diseases to find ingenious ways to pass on their curse.

CHAPTER 12 –
THE MIGHTY MOSQUITO

Some of the greatest sources of infectious human diseases are blood-sucking insects, and globally the most frequent predator is the mosquito. In reality, however, mosquitoes don't cause disease – they are just the unwitting vehicles used by bugs as convenient forms of public transport.

Malaria

"Welcome to Ann … she drinks blood!" started a Second World War US government information leaflet created by the famous educationalist and children's writer Dr Seuss. "Her trade is dishing out malaria. She's at home in Africa, the Caribbean, India, the South and Southwest Pacific and other hot spots. Ann moves around at night (a real party gal) and she's got a thirst. No whiskey, gin, beer or rum coke for Ann … she drinks G.I. blood. She jabs that beak of hers in like a drill and sucks up the juice … then the poor G.I. is going to feel awful in about eight or fourteen days … because he is going to have malaria."

Ann's full name is *Anopheles sp.* She's a type of mosquito, and part of the charm for Dr Seuss as he wrote the leaflet for servicemen, is that it's only female beasts that bite. Ann was portrayed as a wily whore who, if entertained, will give you no end of grief. The mosquito's aim is to get blood, break it down and use it as a food source to mature her eggs. On its own this causes few problems. Just a slight itch as you react to chemicals in the mosquito's saliva designed to stop your blood clotting and help the flow. The last thing a mosquito wants is a clot in its needle-like mouth parts.

The problem is that the saliva is sometimes contaminated. In the case of anopheline mosquitoes the contaminant is all too often one of the malaria plasmodia. While Charles-Louis Laveran got his Nobel Prize for linking malaria with these protozoa, Indian-born Englishman Ronald Ross picked up the 1902 prize for determining that mosquitoes were the infective beast of burden. In one crucial experiment on August 16, 1897, he took ten anopheline mosquitoes that had recently emerged from larvae and introduced them to Husein Khan, a man who was suffering from malaria. The mosquitoes had a good feed, and Khan was paid ten annas for his services. Ross then dissected one or two mosquitoes a day under his microscope. Three days from their feed he found strange looking cells in the mosquitoes' stomachs and on the next two days he found that these cells had grown in size. He realised that he was on the right trail and in excitement penned a poem before retiring to bed that evening.

> This day relenting God
> Hath placed within my hand
> A wondrous thing; and God
> Be praised. At His command,
>
> Seeking His secret deeds
> With tears and toiling breath,
> I find thy cunning seeds,
> O million-murdering Death.
>
> I know this little thing
> A myriad men will save.
> O Death, where is thy sting,
> Thy victory, O grave.[1]

His next breakthrough came in June 1898 when he fed mosquitoes on malaria-infected birds, and then put the insects in a cage with a batch of uninfected birds. The new birds caught malaria. Ross went on to find what he called "germinal rods" in the mosquitoes' stomachs, blood cavity and salivary glands. On July 9 he wrote to his mentor in London saying "I think I may now say QED".

Before this work people thought that malaria came from bad air — mala aria — particularly the sort of stale air that one encounters near swamps. Once Ross had linked the disease to mosquitoes, it proved that the association with swamps was true.

Around the globe there are about three hundred and eighty species of anopheline mosquito, but only sixty or so species are able to transmit the parasite. Like all other mosquitoes, the *Anopheles* breed in water, each species having its preferred breeding grounds, feeding patterns and resting-places. The plasmodia develop in the mosquito's gut and are passed on in the saliva of an infected insect each time it takes a new blood meal. Swept along in the recipient's blood stream, the parasites land up in the liver where they invade the cells and multiply – hundreds become millions.

After about a week, the parasites burst out into the blood stream and penetrate red blood cells. The sudden arrival in the blood stream of masses of parasites plus all the toxic gunk that has built up in the liver cells triggers a fever. Surprisingly, although many diseases cause a person's temperature to rise, no-one knows very much about the mechanism or the purpose. It is clearly a deliberate response by the body, which performs a remarkable *tour de force* in the way that it regulates its temperature.

Fever is not a loss of control, but the body deciding to turn up the thermostat. The signal for this is the release from white blood cells of endogenous pyrogens, a set of small proteins that act on the brain to cause temperature change. As the fever starts there is a discrepancy between the biological mechanisms that measure the person's temperature and those that control it. The consequence is that although his temperature is rising, the person feels cold and shivery. As a result of shivering, wrapping himself up to "keep warm" and some physiological mechanisms that start pumping out heat, his temperature soars to the higher set-point and he no longer feels cold. He may well be totally unaware that his temperature is above normal. As the kidneys clear the toxins from the blood, the fever stimulus is removed. Now the reverse happens. The person feels extremely hot and sweats profusely. Evaporating sweat cools his body until his temperature matches the original set-point.

And why do it? There is some evidence that increasing your temperature makes it harder for the infective agent to survive and increases the immune system's power. Intriguingly, desert iguanas, which can only alter their body temperature by moving in or out of shade, deliberately move into hotter environments when ill. If they are prevented from moving, their mortality rate increases.

I experienced this once while on a business trip in Holland. I had recently returned from a trip to Pakistan and was unaware that I had passengers on-board. I'd flown in from London in the evening, planning to get a good night's sleep and be ready for a course that I was due to teach the next day. But as I went to bed I felt cold. I wasn't too surprised because it was early spring and there was a frost outside, but it was a good hotel and I thought the room should have been warmer. I climbed into bed and pulled two duvets over me. In the middle of the night I woke. Soaked in sweat and feeling sick I fumbled my way to the bathroom and sat perched on the side of the bath facing the loo. I was convinced I had food poisoning, but I wasn't sick and after an hour my temperature felt normal. I felt exhausted and returned to my bed. In the morning I was tired, but able to teach and I only realised the cause of my fever when I saw my doctor a few days later.

What happens next depends on the type of malaria parasite you have been unfortunate enough to pick up. *Plasmodium falciparum* is the one to avoid. Once in a person this moves to the liver and undergoes a thirty thousand-fold multiplication. Breaking out of the liver it enters red blood cells and starts to multiply again. Once every forty-eight hours the newly formed army of bugs bursts from the red blood cells and immediately infects others. If the person can't combat this, the disease escalates every other day. During this process the blood cells become sticky and adhere to capillary walls. Blood flow is reduced. This is particularly nasty when it happens in the brain where it causes a lack of oxygen, coma and death – so-called cerebral malaria.

The mildest form of malaria for humans is *P. malariae*. The replication cycle in the red blood cells is slower, with parasites erupting every seventy-two hours, so the body has more of a chance of dealing with the invaders. The number of bugs floating around in the blood is very low and is easily missed, but they can be there for many years if the person doesn't take appropriate medication.

P. vivax and *P. ovale* can survive and grow at lower temperatures than *P. falciparum* and as a result *P. vivax* has occasionally been transmitted in the UK and the Netherlands. None of the parasites can complete its breeding cycle in temperatures below 15°C.

In rural Africa, people may get bitten several times a night. The consequence is that most babies are exposed to the disease young and suffer severe anaemia. Survivors gradually acquire immunity to their local variant of the disease, so that by adolescence most have got the majority of the parasites out of their system. Adults get the occasional bout of malaria as the body temporarily loses a grip on the situation, and women are particularly prone during their first pregnancy when their immunity seems to fall. Taking a trip to a slightly different area, maybe even just visiting a nearby village, can expose an adult to a novel strain of the disease, and to a new danger. To be safe, you need immunity to each strain. In fact the travellers who are most at risk of the disease are people living in one malaria-infected area, who assume that they are immune, and therefore feel free to travel to another zone without taking preventative medication.

Throwing Up Defences

Knowing the route that a disease uses to move from one person to another is just the first step in combating infection, and the twentieth century saw many attempts to break the human-mosquito-human breeding cycle. If you are wanting a measure of success or failure then consider that three hundred million people worldwide are currently infected by malaria and between one million and one and a half million die from it each year. In 1999 the WHO warned of "a serious risk of uncontrollable resurgence of malaria" in Europe owing to civil disorder, global warming, increased irrigation and international travel.[2]

Get rid of mosquitoes and the disease will disappear. Spraying DDT seemed to be the answer when the insecticide arrived at the end of the Second World War. You could spray the chemical on the walls of your house and for weeks after mosquitoes would drop dead as soon as they landed on the surface and absorbed the poison. Initially this had remarkable effects. In some Greek islands the disease was wiped out for four years. When spraying stopped, a new set of mosquitoes returned, but they had no malaria. Between 1950 and 1970 DDT chased mosquitoes and malaria out of Europe, the United States and Russia. Less of an effort was put into freeing the vast expanses of sub-Saharan Africa. Then mosquitoes learned how to survive DDT, and for that matter many other insecticides, and the eradication programme ground to a halt and was abandoned in 1969. Europe was declared free of malaria in 1975 and as malaria was geographically on the edge of viability the continent has kept clear. Some areas, however, have seen the bug return. In Africa and Asia the disease is endemic.

Global warming could complicate the picture, making more areas available to anopheline mosquitoes and hence to malaria. The general feeling at the moment is that malaria will move to higher areas of ground in countries where it is already endemic, but is unlikely to make a major inroad into new territories. Cities like Harare in the African uplands, which had previously been fairly safe, will lose their freedom from the disease, but regions like mainland Europe should be safe. At least that's what the experts think now.

Drugs that combat malaria are used in two different ways. The first is to try to prevent a person succumbing to an infection. These are taken in acknowledgement of the fact that it is almost impossible to live in or travel to some areas of the world without being bitten by a malaria-bearing mosquito and taking on-board some of the parasites. The idea is that your blood is loaded with parasite-killing drugs so that they die on entry.

The first drug to be used was quinine, an extract from the bark of the South American chinchona tree. This was known to fight off the disease, but at the doses needed it is extremely bitter. Legend has it that the favourite British tipple of gin and tonic started life as a solution to the problem. Mixing quinine with gin and lemon or lime juice made it more palatable. You still find quinine in tonic water, albeit at too low a concentration to have any medicinal value, and the drink got an English patent in 1858 before being bought by Schweppes in 1953. However, synthetic compounds like chloroquine, mefloquine and proguanil have taken over as the mainstay of this prophylaxis.

The second use of the drugs acknowledges that preventative measures often fail, and this time they are employed to wipe out a disease that has become established in a person's body.

Until the 1950s all available anti-malarial drugs worked well. The arrival of chloroquinine resistance in Colombia was a tragic development. Soon it was found on the Thai-Cambodian boarder and reached Africa in the late 1970s. In some areas there is mild resistance and chloroquinine initially knocks the bug back, but after a few days it returns. In other areas, such as Africa, the drug has little or no effect, particularly against *P. falciparum*. This is particularly bad news as chloroquinine is the only inexpensive anti-malarial available in developing countries. Tourists who do use it as a prophylactic need to start taking it a couple of weeks before travelling to build up blood-concentrations of the drug slowly, and continue for some four weeks after they return to eradicate all possible invaders.

Proguanil arrived on the scene at about the same time, but again it wasn't long before some of the parasites had found ways of dealing with it. It is useful, however, when used in combination with other drugs, as multi-resistance that includes this drug is still fairly rare. A standard package is a daily dose of proguanil and weekly chloroquinine.

Multi-drug resistance can develop rapidly as new drugs are introduced and on the Thai-Cambodian border forty per cent of *P. falciparum* cases are also resistant to chloroquinine as well as the more expensive mefloquine. Mefloquine was developed by the American army during the Vietnam war and has been used successfully in Africa. As with so many drugs, the drawback of mefloquine is its side effects. They don't get everyone who takes the tablets, but some people have vivid dreams and nightmares along with attacks of anxiety and depression. The result has been that a few people have returned from their supposedly relaxing holiday in the tropics feeling more stressed than when they left.

Soaking bed nets in insecticide has been a powerful bug-buster. Mosquitoes are attracted to the net by the carbon dioxide breathed out by the sleeping person inside, but die as they land on it. It also means that the nets can be effective even if they have small holes, because the mosquito is still likely to land on the net before finding the hole. This has led to a massive reduction of disease. The insecticide-impregnated nets seem particularly useful in protecting women and babies. Trials organised by the London School of Hygiene and Tropical Medicine, which took place in Burkina Faso, the Gambia, Ghana and Kenya show that treated bed nets halved the numbers of children aged six months to four years who die of malaria. There is, however, some concern that preventing babies from getting infected stops them building up immunity, and then they may suffer more severely as adolescents.

Despite these worries, travellers who stay in cities have little to fear in most countries. Leaving cities and heading out into rural areas increases a person's risk of meeting *Anopheles* mosquitoes. Going to an area of jungle or one where jungle has recently been cleared for housing or agriculture makes it a distinct possibility. Forty-eight out of just over four thousand British troops from the First and Second Battalions of the Parachute Regiment sent to Sierra Leone with only one day's notice found out how critical it was to take prophylactic medication. To start with they didn't take the drug for the recommended two weeks prior to departure, and then their supply chain ran out of mefloquine. They contracted malaria.

Anyone who visits malaria-infected regions but takes no precautions exposes himself or herself to a severe risk of catching the disease. However, they do become useful research tools. "Non-immune travellers who are foolish enough to ignore prophylactic measures provide an indication of levels of transmission and risk, rather like canaries that used to be taken down the mines provided an indication of air quality," says malaria expert David Bradley from the London School of Hygiene and Tropical Medicine.[3]

Sometimes help comes from unusual sources. July 2000 saw the Bill and Melinda Gates Foundation donate $40 million toward UK projects aimed at combating malaria. While this is welcome, it is a drop in the ocean of finance that will be needed if the G8 countries are going to realise their desire to see the global burden of malaria reduced by fifty percent by 2010.

Relieving the financial burden of malaria would make a huge difference in poor countries. The WHO claims that people in sub-Saharan Africa spend between £0.03 and £1.40 per person per month on coils, aerosol sprays, treated bed nets and mosquito repellents. This means that a family of five spends £37.00 per year out of an average annual income of £340. To help the situation, Uganda announced in July 2000 that it was removing all taxes from anti-malarial products. In 1999 Tanzania had reduced the sales tax on its products to five per cent, compared to forty-two per cent in countries like Congo and Kenya, with Nigeria and Rwanda making their mosquito nets cost £2.35. This compares to the £30 that you need to pay for a net in Swaziland and £20 in Sudan.

West Nile Encephalitis

Malaria isn't the only headline grabber when it comes to mosquito-borne disease. A relatively recent outbreak of West Nile encephalitis has been getting more than its fair share of the news, not because of the scale of the epidemic, but because of its location – New York City, which has a population of more than eight and a half million people.

On August 23, 1999, an infectious disease consultant from a hospital in Northern Queens district of New York contacted the New York City Department of Health. He had two patients with encephalitis. After a few phone calls the department found four more in other hospitals. Five of them were extremely weak and being kept alive on ventilators.[4] Early tests showed that the cause was an arbo virus – an arthropod-borne virus. The arthropod was almost certainly a mosquito. By September 23, genetic testing of the agent showed that it looked very much like West Nile virus.

By September 28 twenty people had been reported to the CDC and four of them had died. By the end of the autumn the number had risen to sixty cases of the disease, with seven deaths. All the people had come from New York City or its immediate suburbs. Equal numbers of men and women were affected, but older people seemed most prone. Sixty per cent were over the age of sixty-five and the oldest was a ninety-year-old.

Symptoms of the disease are unpleasant to say the least. Three to five days after getting bitten the person develops a high fever and at first probably goes to bed thinking he or she has 'flu. When headaches are joined by a sore throat, backache, muscle pain, joint pain, eyestrain and blurred vision victims get more worried. The appearance of a rash that can cover the whole body normally causes great concern. Anorexia, nausea, vomiting, diarrhoea and breathing difficulties make it a totally unpleasant experience. On top of this one in six people who have the symptoms of the disease can go into a coma and die.

Panic set in. An emergency phone line set up in New York City on September 3 had taken one hundred and thirty thousand calls by the end of the month. That's more than three a minute – day and night. Another twelve thousand calls went to a second hotline set up by the Westchester County Department of Health. Fire stations handed out some three hundred thousand cans of DEET-based mosquito repellent and seven hundred and fifty thousand leaflets advised people about how to minimise their risk. Websites, radio and television broadcasts and local papers went into over-drive urging people to stay indoors in the evenings and wear long-sleeved shirts and long trousers. People were also asked to stay inside while trucks, planes and helicopters sprayed insecticide to rid the place of mosquitoes. Spraying has been likened to shooting at an assailant in the dark, "but at least it gives you something to do," says Dr Vincent Deubel, a virologist at the Pasteur Institute in Paris who has studied West Nile outbreaks for fifteen years.[5]

The first frosts brought welcome relief from not only the disease but also the measures being used to combat it. New Yorkers held their breath as spring 2000 turned into summer. Would the virus have survived the winter?

In July 2000 helicopters took to the air, once more dumping tons of insecticide in an attempt to wipe out mosquitoes. West Nile virus had killed thirty-two birds in and around the city. Two had been found in Manhattan, an area previously unaffected by the virus. A New York Philharmonic concert in Central Park was cancelled after mosquitoes trapped in the area tested positive for the virus. The disease had survived and was back to haunt them. Then, on August 4, the CDC announced that a seventy-eight-year old man on Staten Island had tested positive for West Nile virus. He had become ill on July 22 and went into hospital two days later. Thankfully, he wasn't too badly affected and went home after a week. Then dead birds started showing up in more and more locations. Any hopes that New York and the rest of the United States might get a reprieve were thoroughly dashed.

A survey based on a random sample of people living in the affected area and reported in March 2000 showed the hidden depths of the viral epidemic, but also gave reasons for optimism. "We estimate that approximately 2.6 per cent of persons aged five years and older in the surveyed area in northern Queens were infected with [the virus] but either had no symptoms or experienced mild illness. These findings are not unexpected, and are similar to rates found in a comparable survey following a 1996 outbreak of West Nile encephalitis in Bucharest, Romania," commented New York City health commissioner Neal Cohen.[6] While this shows a high level of previously unrecognised infection, it also suggests that for most people getting a load of the virus doesn't cause any damage – the body is quite capable of fighting it off. "It's horrible for the few individuals who've been terribly affected, but I don't see any way that it will cause more than a dribble of cases [in the US]," says Paul W. Ewald, a biologist at Amherst College who specialises in the history of infectious diseases.[7]

A year after the first person became ill the consequences of the insecticide spraying appeared to be coming to light. Ninety-five per cent of the local lobster population in Long Island Sound, just off the coast of New York, had suddenly died. One of the insecticides used is toxic to lobsters as well as mosquitoes. It is a pyrethroid, and preliminary tests have found traces of it in the lobsters. Its toxic effects mean that it is banned in the UK.[8] The theory is that heavy rains from Hurricane Floyd had washed the poison into drains that feed out to Long Island Sound. One part per billion is enough to kill. It could take a decade for the lobster population to recover.

Virus' Vector

Like malaria parasites, West Nile viruses are moved from person to person by mosquitoes. However, that is where most similarities end. Malaria undergoes vital stages of its life-cycle inside the mosquito, but for West Nile virus the insect is a simple airborne vehicle. Because of this development process, malaria is confined to the *Anopheles* mosquito, but West Nile virus is free to use at least forty-three different species including *Anopheles*, *Culex* and *Aedes* mosquitoes.

In addition, the type of malaria that infects humans has no other animal reservoir. *Anopheles* mosquitoes may draw blood from a wide range of animals, but only when they bite infected human beings do they pick up human malaria. In contrast, West Nile virus is at home in a variety of animals including horses and birds. Dogs and cats seem to be immune. In fact, the first clues to the nature of the virus came from the Bronx Zoo where twenty flamingos, herons and bald eagles suddenly died at about the same time as the first human cases were reported. At the time, health experts were considering whether they had St Louis encephalitis on their hands. Birds, however, are known to be immune to that bug, so clearly another agent was at large.

The main vector for West Nile virus is the *Culex* mosquito, a type that is at home in cities. It's quite happy to breed in a discarded can or bottle, a pond, puddle or garden water butt. Again, piles of old tyres that collect small pockets of water when left out in the rain are favourite dwelling places and a prime source of mosquito production. Government advice includes drilling holes in the sides of old tyres so that water can't accumulate and covering any piles with waterproof sheets. Much of the New York publicity campaign has been targeted at getting people to fill in puddles and clear debris from their roof gutters so that no pool of water can collect in them and emptying garden paddling pools when they are not in use. Even garden birdbaths have come in for attention, with owners asked to clean them out every two or three days.

It takes about a week to ten days from the time a mosquito feeds on an infected person or animal until the virus shows up in the insect's saliva. Only when this happens is the critter infective.

Point of Origin

New York's outbreak of West Nile virus shows just how easily diseases that are classically thought of as being confined to one area of the world or another can jump ship. The virus was first isolated in the West Nile district of Uganda in 1937, but it wasn't long before people realised it was the most widespread member of the group of flaviviruses. It has been found throughout Europe, Africa and Eurasia. Australia and Southeast Asia have Kunjin virus, their own variation on the theme.

An outbreak of West Nile fever in Israel in 1950 caused five hundred clinical cases, and epidemics happened in 1951, 1952, 1953 and 1957. In each year the zone affected by the disease was very small. Between 1962–65 and 1975–80 there were outbreaks in France and the largest recorded epidemic occurred in 1974 in South Africa, when there were thousands of clinical cases of West Nile encephalitis.

The mechanism by which it moved across the Atlantic Ocean to New York remains a mystery. It's possible that the disease has been around for a few years, but because most people don't get ill, it has simply gone unnoticed. On the other hand, a newly-infected human could have caught a plane and travelled from Africa or Eastern Europe arriving at a New York City airport just as the virus levels in his blood peaked. A bite or two from a mosquito moved the virus to local birds where the virus multiplied.

By summer 2000 it was clear that the virus was almost identical to a strain of West Nile virus found in a goose on an Israeli farm. With tens of thousands of passengers travelling each year between New York and the Middle East, this seems the most likely source. Between July 1998 and June 1999, five million people arrived in the New York area planning to stay there at least a few days. Of these, 2.1 million had come from places known to contain West Nile viruses.

Another possibility is that the virus entered America in an infected bird. It could have flown there as part of its migratory route, or been imported, either legally or illegally, into the country as a pet, zoo exhibit or laboratory animal. It is always possible that the introduction was a deliberate act of biological terrorism.

Regardless of its source and mode of entry, West Nile virus is now part of the US ecological environment. It has proved that it is capable of surviving one winter and there are reports of it moving to other parts of the East Coast. "We're beyond containment now," comments Robert G. McLean, a US government biologist studying West Nile's impact on birds. "We have to live with it and do the best we can." New York State's wildlife pathologist Ward Stone said, "It will become one of the diseases in America that we have to watch for. And we should be getting ready for the next one."⁹

Maybe the arrival of this disease in the most expensive region of America will stimulate the release of funds to take a serious look at removing mosquitoes by more intelligent means than bombing them with chemicals. If so it could do a great favour to the rest of the world as the spin-off could be enhanced measures to tackle other mosquito-transmitted diseases, such as malaria.

Yellow Fever

Mosquitoes also play a large role in Yellow Fever. It's a disease that probably originated in Africa, but found its way into the Americas via the slave trade. The disease is caused by another flavivirus that makes use of the *Aedes aegypti* mosquito. As well as passing the disease on by biting infected people, the mosquito can pass it on to future generations of insects as the virus moves into its eggs. The eggs can lie dormant in a dried-up riverbed waiting for the rainy season and the right opportunity to spring to life. Newly-emerged mosquitoes come with built-in killing power, moving the disease into a new season of horror.

Yellow Fever also has a strong hold in monkeys. As a result, living near a jungle, or travelling to one, exposes you to the risk of picking the disease up from mosquitoes that have fed on an ape at some time in the past.

Young men working as loggers in forests are particularly prone to this route of infection. Urban outbreaks of Yellow Fever happen when an infected person goes into a city. Domestic mosquitoes, of which *Aedes aegypti* is an example, soon spread the virus. The effect can be an outbreak that has a clear epicentre, but spreads rapidly across a wide area.

These two mechanisms of catching and spreading the disease come about because of economic pressures and life-style. One drives people into forests to work, or causes shantytowns to develop on the edge of recently deforested land, the other is a feature of urbanisation. Each mosquito can only travel a few hundred feet, so to cause an epidemic it needs to encounter plenty of people in that small zone. Mega-cities give it all the possibilities it needs.

Yellow Fever is a gruesome disease. The virus incubates silently for three to six days after entering a person's blood stream. Then fever sets in accompanied by muscle pain, headaches, shivers, loss of appetite and nausea – with or without vomiting. And that's the mild part of the disease. Thankfully, seven out of eight do not progress to the nasty part and get toxic shock. For the rest, after a twenty-four hour break from the suffering the fever returns with a vengeance, and the person turns yellow with jaundice – hence its name – and complains of stomach pains. Victims start to bleed from the mouth, nose, eyes and stomach. Blood appears in vomit and faeces. The kidneys fail to cope and half the people who reach this stage die within twelve to fourteen days. The other half recover to tell the tale.

This is a disease that has caused great suffering, but from time to time in recent history we have had it on the run. In 1793 it killed five thousand people in Philadelphia and in 1798 two to three thousand people fell to its spell in New York. An eradication program set up by the Rockefeller Foundation in 1915 started to address the issue. In particular, the Foundation was keen to prevent Yellow Fever from passing through the recently opened Panama Canal and on to Asia. In 1947 the disease was driven out of North America. Mexico, Central America and most of South America were free by 1970. At that point the programme was wound down, and the mosquitoes and the disease have crept back.

In addition there is a good vaccine, but not everyone who needs it gets it. Over three hundred million doses of this live virus vaccine have been given around the world, with side effects almost solely confined to children under the age of six months. Consequently, it is now given only to older children and adults. The WHO strongly recommends childhood vaccination at about nine months. A single dose gives at least ten years' protection.

Between 1939 and 1952 vaccination all but eradicated Yellow Fever from French West Africa. Gambia had an epidemic of the disease in 1979–80 and instigated a programme of mass vaccination. By 1997 they had achieved ninety-one per cent coverage, and no cases of Yellow Fever have occurred since. Nearby in Mali only one per cent of the population has received the vaccine. One of the problems is the cost of vaccination. Each dose costs the equivalent of £0.12/US $0.18, a heavy burden for some of these struggling nations. Yet the virus remains, lurking in the background, so any let-up in the vaccination strategy would see a rapid return of the scourge.

Indeed, over the last two decades of the twentieth century, most African countries saw increasing numbers of victims. In 1985 there were around one thousand but by 1991 this had soared to five thousand. And these are the reported numbers. The WHO believes that this may represent as little as half of one per cent of the true scale of disease. The increase is blamed on the standard factors – increasing numbers of mosquitoes, deforestation, urbanisation and widespread international travel.

Other Possibilities

It is worth pointing out that mosquitoes can't transmit HIV. When HIV-AIDS first came on the scene it was a great cause for concern, but one that thankfully has now receded. To start with, mosquitoes digest HIV. Any virus that got taken up by a feeding mosquito would be broken down within one to two days, so wouldn't be around when the female mosquito needs to feed again to mature the next batch of her eggs. In addition, it seems unlikely that a mosquito would ingest many HIV particles at a feed. This is because HIV is not present in particularly high concentrations in blood. Take, for example, a mosquito that was feeding on an HIV-infected person with a concentration of particles one hundred times higher than usual. Interrupt it mid-feed and place it straight on to an HIV-free individual so that it can finish its meal. Scientists calculate that even in this extreme situation, there is only a one-in-ten-million chance of getting an infective dose.

Mosquitoes' mouth parts are supremely complex. They are designed to deliver saliva through one tube and draw blood through another. This means that for a virus to leave the mosquito it has to travel from the insect's stomach into its salivary glands. This is a feat that HIV can't achieve. So far, it appears we are safe from this peril.

While we can be relieved about HIV, there is some evidence that hepatitis C might be moved around by mosquitoes. Presenting data at a microbiology meeting in Los Angeles in May 2000, Dominique Debriel and colleagues from the Hospital Pasteur in Grenoble, France, showed that the hepatitis C virus was quite capable of living inside mosquito cells. She stressed, however, that the work was preliminary saying, "The most I can say is that this is the first evidence that mosquito cells can bind and replicate the virus."[10] However, the implication of the data is that hepatitis C may be about to join the list of diseases known to be spread by these versatile insects.

CHAPTER 13 -
FOOT-AND-MOUTH

You will probably never have the opportunity, but if you do, try this. Lean gently over a British livestock farmer just as he is going to sleep and whisper "Little Warley" or "Heddon-on-the-Wall" into his ear. It is liable to induce nightmares. Similarly start a conversation on the subject of culls or mass slaughter and you are likely to invoke an involuntary grimace as his senses recall the sight, sound and stench of raging funeral pyres. For that matter, mentioning the year 2001 will probably have a similar effect for the rest of his life.

The reason for this is foot-and-mouth. It took eight months from the time when the first animals were identified to the point that a whole week went by without a fresh outbreak and by then the statistics of the destruction were staggering. Mass death had visited more than 9,500 farms destroying over 3.9 million cattle, sheep, pigs, goats and deer. Estimates of the full cost of the epidemic range from £3 billion to £3.5 billion and there was talk of taxes having to rise to help the British government pick up its part of the bill.

I include foot-and-mouth in the book, not because it infects humans, but because it is the most vivid example of an economic disease – a disease that damages, sometimes even decimates, aspects of a country's trade. It is also a clear case-history of how difficult it is to eradicate a disease once it has got out into a general population.

The first indication that Britain had a problem came on February 19, 2001 when an observant vet became anxious. He was performing a routine check on the health of a batch of 720 pigs that were waiting in a holding pen within a slaughterhouse owned by Cheale Meats just outside Little Warley, a village in the north east of England. Twenty-eight of the pigs were lying down and looked lethargic, both signs of ill-health. When he saw blisters on the flesh next to the hard part of their hooves and on their lips, gums and tongue he triggered a chain reaction that set alarm bells ringing around the world. They are symptoms of a number of different diseases, one of which is foot-and-mouth disease, which is so feared amongst farming folk that many countries ban all imports of livestock and meat from countries where it is known to exist.

This particular slaughterhouse is a busy outfit that takes animals from around Britain and distributes the meat around Europe. Once lab tests showed that the disease was indeed foot-and-mouth, the question in everyone's mind was, "how big is this epidemic?" Commentators were quick to start to draw comparisons with the previous outbreak in 1967–68 that visited 2,364 farms across Britain and was brought under control by the slaughter of 442,000 animals. Dr Alex Donaldson, head of the UK's major centre for studying foot-and-mouth disease, the Pirbright Laboratory at the Institute of Animal Health, told reporters on the first day of the outbreak that he hoped the outbreak would be nothing like that, "At the moment there's just one officially recorded outbreak, but we really don't know what the future holds." Too right.

It turns out that the disease had been present in the UK for at least a couple of weeks, and that the index case – the initial site of the outbreak – was in a farm hundreds of miles away from the slaughterhouse.

The Anatomy of the Disease

Foot-and-mouth affects all cloven-hoofed animals and disease experts say that it is the most contagious of all animal diseases. An infection can be triggered by the animal receiving as few as ten of the disease-causing viruses. Far from being a gruesome killer, foot-and-mouth results in a relatively minor disease and seldom kills the animals that meet the virus. Infected animals have a short-lived fever and get blisters chiefly in the mouth and on the feet. Most recover within a couple of weeks without any treatment. There are some types of animals that are more vulnerable such as suckling pigs, but the majority suffer from an illness that is just about as unpleasant as a common cold, or a mild case of 'flu.

The problem with the disease is less what it does to the animals, than what it does to the bank-balance of the owner. While the virus causes only mild discomfort to the farmer's livestock it causes considerable pain to his finances. "Foot-and-mouth is the most economically important single livestock disease worldwide and perhaps the most contagious," claims Harley Moon, one time director of the US Department of Agriculture's Plum Island Animal Disease Center, near New York. It is the world's best example of an economic-killer-germ. The problem is that an animal infected by foot-and-mouth becomes less productive. Its milk production drops and its ability to grow – and therefore to put on meat – is reduced. In the world of agri-business that loss of efficiency in the livestock is an offence worthy of capital punishment. It will not be tolerated.

Intriguingly there are no real figures that demonstrate the true extent of the damage to productivity that foot-and-mouth can wreak on a group of animals, because, as veterinary historian working at the University of Manchester Abigail Woods, explains, since the 1920s no animal with the disease has been allowed to live – any animal infected with the disease is immediately slaughtered.

Foot-and-mouth is particularly difficult to control because infected animals pump out millions of viruses each hour for days before clinical signs appear. Scientists classify the virus as a *Picornaviridae*, genus *Aphthovirus* – it is the same family as the virus that causes polio. So far scientists have identified seven broad types called serotypes (O, A, C, SAT1, SAT2, SAT3 and Asia 1) and the 2001 UK outbreak was caused by a version known as pan-Asiatic serotype O.

The virus grows predominantly in an animal's gut and is excreted in vast numbers in faeces. Consequently, water contamination is a problem as rain-water and washings run from farmyards and fields into ditches, streams and rivers, carrying the virus rapidly to new areas. Animal transport is another cause for concern as liquid and muck dropping from livestock trucks can trail a web of disease around an entire country as the vehicle criss-crosses it visiting numerous farms, markets and abattoirs as part of its normal weekly routine.

The tell-tale blisters also play their part in transmission. Each fluid-filled bulge is packed with high concentrations of the virus. As the blisters burst and the animals cough, clouds of viruses take to the air. Borne on winds they may travel vast distances. Circumstantial evidence indicates that a 1981 outbreak of the disease on the Isle of Wight, just south of the British mainland, was caused by the virus having blown over the English Channel from infected animals on the north coast of France, 60 or more miles (96 kilometres) away.

The other point of concern is that the virus can live on in an animal's meat and milk if they are not treated properly. After killing an animal, carcasses are normally hung in a cool room for them to cure. Part of the process that follows involves the meat becoming very slightly acidic. This change in the nature of the meat is enough to destroy most of the viruses, but some remain. Consequently, when food waste is fed to pigs in the form of pig-swill, there are strict rules about the need to boil the swill for long periods to ensure that any remaining viruses do not survive. In a similar way, any viruses that make their way into an animal's milk are effectively removed by the heat treatment used to pasteurise it. Distributing untreated milk is one way of spreading the disease.

The general wisdom is that cattle are mainly infected by inhalation of the viruses – often from pigs, while pigs are mainly infected by ingesting contaminated food and expelling large amounts of virus in respiratory aerosols. Sheep form a particular problem in that when they become infected the disease causes only mild symptoms — symptoms that are easily missed. They can therefore provide a safe harbour for the viruses and if the sheep are moved from farm to farm then the virus goes along too.

It takes anything from two to twenty-one days from the point when an animal meets the virus to the time that symptoms start to appear, although in most cases they show in three to eight days. One of the problems in leaving the disease to run its course is that while the animals recover quickly they still have active viruses on-board and continue to excrete them for anything up to two months in the case of sheep, or two years in cattle.

Farm animals are not the only culprits when it comes to spreading the disease. People do the job very well. A walker who steps in an infected cow pat will deposit the virus with each footfall for the rest of his or her walk. So too the dog that he or she is exercising can transport the virus attached to feet or fur. Birds have a great opportunity to move between farms, and although most are highly territorial and don't range far, they form an inter-linking set of connections that are capable of speedily carrying the virus from the centre of an outbreak to surrounding premises. Wild deer form an obvious vehicle. As cloven-hoofed animals they are susceptible to the disease so they can theoretically not only act as transports, but also amplify the numbers of viruses as they go. While their roaming is fairly confined, it is quite sufficient to move the disease between adjacent farms.

And while we are drawing up our list of villains, it is vitally important not to forget other members of the farming industry. Vets who travel from farm to farm are ideal transporters of disease. So are lorries delivering feed or collecting milk and other produce, unless the farm is arranged so that they are loaded and unloaded while still on the road and don't actually come onto the premises. Then there is the farmer. With the reduction in the number of personnel working in agriculture, individual farmers now frequently run a number of different farms. They are in a great position to distribute disease over a wide area if it starts up on one of their businesses.

Add to this the fact that many farms have made their permanent staff redundant and instead use contractors who chase from farm to farm. Don't forget that many farms are also family homes and cannot be isolated in the way that you would isolate an industrial site.

Can Foot-and-Mouth Infect Humans?

The evidence that foot-and-mouth can infect humans is sparse. In the 1966–67 UK outbreak thirty-five-year-old Bobby Brewis rose to fame when he caught the disease. He worked as a farm machinery salesman and lived on a farm with his brother in Yetlington, a hamlet in Northumberland. The disease broke out on his farm on July 28 and Bobby stood by watching as the animals were slaughtered. He took no part in the operation but may have drunk some unpasteurised milk. Four days later he developed a mild temperature and a sore throat. On top of this he had blisters on the palms of his hands and swellings on his tongue that lasted for a couple of weeks and then went away. It appeared he had foot-and-mouth.

One of the earliest clearly recorded instances of humans getting the disease was in 1834 when three veterinarians deliberately drank raw milk from infected cows, and since then a total of forty people around the world have been diagnosed with the disease.

For a few days it appeared as if viruses from the 2001 outbreak had taken up residence in another human. In mid-April father-of-two Paul Stamper was working culling animals and disposing of carcasses in north Cumbria when one of the carcasses he was about to pick up exploded in his face and some of the fluid splashed into his mouth – and he swallowed. It's enough to make anyone feel sick, but a few days later he had a sore throat and blisters on the back of his throat. He didn't, however, have any on his hands and feet. The unions started complaining about lack of protection for their members and the level of anxiety about the disease went up another notch, but by the end of the month laboratory tests showed that Stamper's disease was no more than an ordinary sore throat. Thirteen other suspected cases came and went the same way.

Once again foot-and-mouth showed that it was almost incapable of crossing the species barrier and infecting humans, though that did not preventing it harming their wallets.

Global History

It is difficult to establish where foot-and-mouth first appeared in the world. "Why?" asks Woods, before answering the question herself. "Because the symptoms are so mild." That said, the first recorded incidence in North America was in 1825, when an article in *American Farmer* magazine talked of farmers finding animals that were becoming lame because the fleshy area between the two parts of their hooves were "sore entirely through" and in the opinion of the farmers, "the disease was clearly contagious."

It was first recorded within the UK in 1839 when it is assumed that the virus came in via live imports of animals, meat or skins, or even on fodder hay. For the rest of the nineteenth-century it was just a part of farming life. Sometimes your stock was fully healthy, at other times it was a little unwell. That was the way things were.

It was only as some farms started to become businesses and breed pedigree animals that anyone really took foot-and-mouth seriously. In 1869 some of these farmers started finding that their more carefully bred animals were more susceptible to the disease and tended to die if infected. Being wealthy they had influence and started to protect their herds by isolating infected farms, closing livestock markets and banning live imports from any country where there was suspicion of disease. It was the start of a policy that would come back to bite the UK.

By the turn of the century the policy appeared to have paid off and Britain was free of the disease. That was until it broke out again in 1920. The disease caught the authorities unprepared and they were soon far behind on the programme of slaughter that was instigated to tackle the disease. In fact they were so far behind that by the time workers showed up on an infected farm to clear out the stock most of the animals had recovered and the agricultural community was beginning to ask what all the fuss was about.

After discussion, the authorities decided to maintain their policy of keeping Britain disease-free and in the 1950s they were successful in encouraging first European countries and then many through the rest of the world to aim for disease-free status. Now the Paris-based Office International des Epizooties keeps a list of the "FMD free countries where vaccination is not practised". Being on the list is valuable because it forms a trading community whose members buy and sell meat and livestock to each other. If you are not on the list you can't trade. The 1990–91 session of the European Community decided on a policy of non-vaccination so that member states could open their borders to free trade in livestock and meat. Ironically the UK, the champion of the system has just been removed from the list.

UK 2001

A brief review of the 2001 outbreak in the UK shows how quickly a disease can take hold and how difficult it is to eradicate. All you need is a system that is not prepared for its arrival, and a collective memory that seems to have forgotten that rapidly spreading diseases have not been confined to history.

While the disease was first spotted on the February 19, this was most certainly not the first day that the virus was in the UK. One of the most likely explanations for the explosion of disease starts with the theory that it arose weeks earlier on a pig farm in Heddon-on-the-Wall, a village in the north east of England. Without anyone being aware that the virus was present there was nothing to stop it spreading and animals held in seven local farms became infected.

Sheep from one of these farms were sent to the nearby Hexham market. They were bought and moved to Longtown on the other side of the country, not to a farm, but to another market. Over the following ten days these sheep were transported and traded around the country, coming into contact with tens of thousands of other animals and passing on the virus at each encounter. The farming system that uses animals as commodities for trade and barter became its own worst enemy.

Tracing the movements of animals became a mammoth task because of the vast number involved. Many of the movements will never be known because inspectors soon found that many sheep had been traded on the outskirts of markets and the sales had never been officially recorded. Finding where any animals were that could have come in contact with infected stock was vital though if there was going to be any hope of putting an early end to the epidemic.

An export ban came into force on February 21, but keen not to over-react the Ministry of Agriculture, Fisheries and Food (MAFF) waited until February 23 before imposing a ban on the movement of all livestock within Britain.

Sadly, between the time the disease entered Britain and this issuing of a movement ban it is estimated that up to two million sheep movements had occurred around the country. The cat was most decidedly out of the bag. Importing countries were anxious to realise that 30,000 sheep had left the country and were mingling with animals across Europe.

An outbreak in Highampton in the south-west corner of the country showed the scale of the problem. On February 25, cattle and sheep from one farm were found to have the disease. The owner of this farm had bought some animals at the Longtown market and inadvertently given a free ride to the disease as he transported them from one end of the country to the other. The trouble was that he also ran 13 other premises and soon the disease was found on many of those.

By February 27 there had been twenty confirmed cases of the disease spread across much of England. Exported sheep in France had been found with the disease and 700 sheep and 1,000 pigs imported to North Rhein-Westphalia in Germany were slaughtered.

By April the situation had deteriorated into a disaster. In the week ending April 17, 1,366 new outbreaks were confirmed. The Army had been called in and teams of slaughtermen were killing and burying tens of thousands of animals a day. The policy was that when a vet suspected that there was an infected animal on a farm all the animals on that farm would be killed. The target was that this destruction should occur within twenty-four hours of the detection. With the animals dead, the viruses couldn't multiply. Rapid slaughter should stop the epidemic in its tracks.

In case the virus had already spread to surrounding farms, all animals on any farm that had a field bordering the infected premises were also slaughtered. It became known as the "contiguous cull".

Killing this number of animals is one thing. Disposing of their carcasses was quite another. The initial scheme of building massive mounds of railway sleepers and coal, and then balancing carcasses on top and igniting the lot was unable to keep up with the flow. In any case there was anxiety that the virus might spread in the smoke and that the pyres might pour toxic fumes into the atmosphere.

The government turned to its disused Second World War airfields. The fields had witnessed one battle before and now they would take part in another. As quickly as earth-moving vehicles carved 150 metre (164-foot) long, 4-metre (13½-foot) deep trenches in the ground, lorries tipped mounds of partially decaying animals in. Bulldozers then pushed earth back over as if trying to hide the evidence. One site in Cumbria had 20 such trenches – enough to accommodate half a million carcasses. Workers and news reporters allowed into the area, spoke of blocks of a hundred or more decomposing sheep thudding into the bottom of the pit, limbs flapping and oozing yellow slimy liquid. Unsurprisingly, a stench of death hung over the site.

As massive pyres started burning up carcasses the British Prime Minister Tony Blair described the situation as "grave" – not I'm sure intended as a pun. But then it was not only the farmers' lives that were being disrupted by the virus. Blair, it was widely assumed, had been gearing up for a General Election in the early summer, probably on May 3. With much of the countryside at a standstill and the government's credibility taking a knocking over indecision about how to fight the disease, this was looking like a bad time to ask the country for permission to have another five years in office. After considerable delay and speculation the election was eventually scheduled for June 7, a date by which Blair hoped that foot-and-mouth would again be cast into history books. He was wrong.

To Cull, to Vaccinate or to Vacillate?

Commentators started looking to the long-term consequences of eradicating the disease by wiping out the animals. Many of the sheep in Cumbria live on fells, open moors that stretch over ancient, granite mountains. The fells are not fenced and the animals need no constraint because they know their place. Each so-called "hefted" sheep lives in the location it was born in. It was born there because that was where its mother was born, and she because her mother had been born in the same area a few years earlier. The pattern repeats back into history. Kill these animals and you wipe out years of heritage, years of learning. Kill these animals and it is difficult to see how modern agriculture will cope with the tiresome task of re-seeding the fells with flocks. Kill these animals and you kill the agriculture that has been practised for years.

There is an alternative to culling if you want to contain disease and that is vaccination. The science is well-known, but it is not one hundred per cent effective for two reasons. First, not all animals that you give the vaccine to will develop an immunity to the disease. Secondly, there is a time lag of days or weeks between giving the vaccine and the animals gaining immunity. It is, of course, frequently used to limit the spread of human diseases because culling is not an option.

Vaccination however has a third problem when it comes to foot-and-mouth. An animal that has been vaccinated can still harbour viruses without showing any signs of the disease. These viruses can be passed on to other unvaccinated stock. For this reason the *cordon sanitaire* that has been established by countries seeking to keep foot-and-mouth out of their fields includes a stipulation that countries wanting to prove they have a clean bill of health must not vaccinate their stock. Consequently you may reduce or even eliminate the effects of the virus, but you cannot participate in international trading of the livestock or meat.

One voice repeatedly called for vaccination. Dr Fred Brown had been the key scientist working on foot-and-mouth in the UK for decades and had left the country to work at the Plum Island research unit in the USA. He was convinced that vaccination would bring the epidemic under control without having to resort to the mass annihilation of the UK herd. Furthermore he was adamant that new tests that he and colleagues had developed were quite capable of detecting whether a vaccinated animal was also harbouring the virus.

Vaccines are based on the virus that causes the disease. The idea is that you expose the animal to a little of the killer germ and allow its immune system to build a defence against it. The vaccine uses viruses that have been effectively tamed so that they look similar, but don't trigger disease. When the animal encounters a wild version of the virus the immune system is primed, ready and waiting. The problem is finding a test that can distinguish between the wild disease-causing virus and the vaccine. Brown's test relies on the fact that wild foot-and-mouth disease viruses produce a particular protein as part of their lifecycle. When the virus is ready to move on to a new host it leaves this protein behind. This protein, however, is not produced by the viruses present in the vaccine. The protein therefore acts as a clear marker of a viral attack, and if the authorities wanted they could use a test to look for it before exporting any animals.

Almost inevitably the summer and autumn saw publications of claims and counter claims arguing for or against each policy. Somewhere at the fringe of the debate was a surprisingly quiet voice of animal rights protesters and Green activists who were appalled at the mass destruction of basically healthy animals for the sole purpose of maintaining an ability to sell animals to countries that by-and-large are quite capable of growing enough of their own. There was something deeply hideous about living in a world where people die of starvation, but at the same time one country can destroy three million farm animals in order to satisfy trade regulations.

Academics working in Britain and Canada built computer models that enabled them to model the spread of disease and concluded that culling was the most effective way of bringing the disease under control. Part of the assumption behind the model was that a vaccination programme would take longer to get in place than slaughter.

One thing however was clear. Cull or vaccinate, the key issue is to move hard and fast as soon as the first case is detected. Any delay in the early stages of the disease allows it to spread and creates a massive pool of disease throughout the country.

Someone to Blame

As with many tragedies people look for someone to blame. It helps people feel slightly better if they can identify the source of their grief and by determining that someone else was responsible they can absolve themselves of guilt.

In reality it is unlikely that the ultimate source of the virus will ever be known – not with certainty. The high probability was that illegally imported meat was used in the kitchens of restaurants in the north east of England and then passed on to farmers who failed to treat it properly before feeding it to their stock.

But that doesn't solve the issue. The particular strain of the disease is unusual and previously unknown in Europe. Similar versions were first identified in Asia a decade ago and have been circulating since.

According to Abigail Woods, in the past it has always been easy to blame Argentine meat, which probably accounted for sixty per cent of disease in the nineteenth century – where the other forty per cent were from they didn't know. Once again a finger of suspicion points at Argentina which claims that it had suffered no outbreaks of the disease in the twelve months preceding the outbreak in the UK. Independent observers have differing views, claiming that Argentine ranchers reportedly burnt at least 3,500 cattle in 2000 after saying that foot-and-mouth disease had spread into ranches from Brazil and Paraguay. While the Argentine government continues to deny the disease, farmers reported three hundred cases of foot-and-mouth in the week that the UK outbreak started.

With the disease being endemic in other parts of the world there is no reason why the virus couldn't have hitched a lift in a traveller's suitcase or backpack.

Then there are the more extreme theories. Dr Harash Narang spent thirty years working in the UK government's public health laboratory. He is convinced that a likely source of the epidemic was an accidental release of the virus from the Pirbright laboratory just south of Oxford, UK, that works on developing and testing vaccines for foot-and-mouth. Of course the laboratory denies this, but human error is always possible.

An even more sensational suggestion was presented at a June 2001 meeting of terrorism experts in Edinburgh. Professor Malcolm Dando, of Bradford University's Department of Peace Studies said that, "Foot-and-mouth is one of the obvious agents you would use if you wanted to attack a country's animal stock. It has been taken very seriously as a possible weapon since the 1940s."

To the Future

As the dust started to settle on this particular outbreak people started to ask questions. Despite calls for a public enquiry the UK government decided to set up three, small enquiries that would meet behind closed doors. The feeling was that they were reluctant for errors to be made public.

Other bodies have decided to join in the fray and set up enquiries of their own. In October 2001 Devon County Council set up a public enquiry chaired by a local resident Professor Ian Mercer. The aim was to find out why their area was so traumatically affected by the disease and to see if this could teach them how to tackle a similar outbreak in the future. The council also wanted to use the opportunity to discuss the future of farming in the UK.

The Devon enquiry concluded that there was a need to increase the import controls if we were going to remove effectively the passports from disease organisms, and that all movements of animals should be banned on the first day an outbreak of a disease like foot-and-mouth is suspected. The recent escalation in the transport of farm animals must be reversed. The report called for a re-appraisal of vaccination for foot-and-mouth and questioned the policy of large-scale burial sites or funeral pyres, echoing the feeling that burning carcasses was "barbaric and medieval". In short the enquiry criticised every aspect of policy and procedure – no wonder the government was keen to hold its own investigation behind closed doors.

The Royal Society, a body of some of the most prominent UK scientists, also set up a public enquiry. Chaired by Professor Sir Brian Follett this committee took a wider remit and looked not only at foot-and-mouth but at a range of other infectious diseases that affect agriculture.

These enquiries are set against a background of a general opinion that the public, and quite possibly the farming and veterinary professions, will not tolerate a mass cull being used as the method of containing disease in the future. Some other strategy needs to be found.

Even without the public enquiry coming to any conclusions there are some interesting lessons that can be learned by comparing statistics from the 1967–68 outbreak with that in 2001. The critical statistics show the pace at which the disease took hold. In 1967–68 the outbreak was abolished by destroying some 434,000 over a period of thirty-two weeks. In 2001 over 2,382,000 animals were slaughtered in the first eleven weeks after the disease was discovered. One of the most pressing questions is how the infection spread so far so fast.

The answers seem to point to changes in agricultural practice in the years in between. In terms of total numbers, Britain has seen relatively little change – a fifty per cent increase in sheep and lamb numbers (20 million in 1967 compared to 30 million in 1999), a twenty per cent decline in cattle (9 million compared to 7.5 million) and a stable level of pig production (about 5 million at both dates). More critically, over this period the number of animals on any one farm has substantially increased. Average sheep flocks have doubled in size from 250 to 510, cattle herds have increased from fifty to ninety and pig production has moved to industrial scales as the average herd has risen from eighty to just under 600. The result of this is that if an infection gets onto a farm it can spread to a large number of animals very easily and any policy based on eradicating all the livestock on a farm if one is found to be infected has a much more drastic effect.

The other intriguing difference is the extent to which animals are transported around the country, and for that matter around the continent and the world. The 1967–68 outbreak was triggered by the virus arriving in a consignment of Argentine lamb and the Ministry of Agriculture attributed all but one of the subsequent 2,364 outbreaks to wind-borne distribution of the virus. The effectiveness of this process was enhanced because the lambs had been placed in the middle of one of the highest concentrations of livestock in the world. High stocking-densities are great for propagating disease. While the local area was badly affected, the disease was contained because no animal movements were allowed.

This was not a huge problem because the agricultural system was not based on moving animals large distances. Short journeys were partly enabled by the fact that there were large numbers of small slaughterhouses around the country. In post-BSE Britain most of the small abattoirs have closed, so animals now travel long distances to meet their slaughterman. In addition, agribusiness has joined many wide-spread farms together, so that animals are frequently moved large distances in order to find fresh pasture.

As a consequence the MAFF (now DEFRA) believe that in 2001 animal movements caused at least ninety-two separate centres of the disease – a stark contrast to the one movement-related case in 1967–8.

The 2001 outbreak of foot-and-mouth disease should act as a wake-up call. It shows the farming industry that it needs to adopt practices that recognise the constant threat of infections. It may decide to adopt vaccination as opposed to culling, but the next outbreak may be a disease that does kill its stock.

It should also form an object lesson to all those working in public health and disease control. High rates of movement combined with high population densities are just what killer germs like best. Once an outbreak is established the first few hours and days are critical. Get the containment right then, and you stand a chance. Wait around trying to work out what is the best policy to pursue and you will have lost the war.

Any policy changes, however, will need to be made on an international basis, because as epidemiologist Professor Mark Woolhouse of Edinburgh University commented in the middle of the outbreak, "We don't just live in a global village, we live on a global farm."[1]

CHAPTER 14 - HEALTHCARE-ACQUIRED INFECTIONS

I've always quipped that you need to be very well before going into hospital. The place is so full of disease-ridden people that you need all your built-in, bug-busting biology to be running at full steam to have a chance of coming out alive. Now I've seen the statistics, I realise that my quip was much more than a joke.

According to UK government figures, around one in ten patients who go into a hospital pick up an infection while they are there. This leads to 100,000 people being infected each year, of whom five thousand die as a direct result of that infection. Think about it for a moment. That is the equivalent of a Boeing 747 crashing once a month and killing all on board. And that's not all. Infections picked up while visiting some form of healthcare provider are one of the causes behind a further 15,000 deaths[1] – now we are up to four 747s a month. And it's a worldwide issue. In the USA, two million people a year get an infection while they are in hospital, and up to 90,000 of these patients die from those infections. The health cost alone is estimated at between $5 billion and $28 billion.

Look at the mechanics of the problem, and it is easy to spot where the increased cost comes from. Getting a bacterial infection in the blood-stream, bacteraemia, causes a person to have to stay in hospital for around eleven extra days. In the USA this adds some $57,000 to the bill for that visit alone. The attention given to this by the average person wandering through a hospital door is surprisingly slight, given that more people die in the USA from hospital-acquired infections than in car accidents and homicides combined.

A survey published in 1999 looked at all of the hospitals in one administrative area of the UK over a thirteen-month period. The findings agreed with the American data, and showed that patients stayed in hospital on average eleven days longer if they picked up an infection, which made their stay two-and-a-half times longer than it would otherwise have been. The UK researchers calculated that even in 1999 this would add over

£2,900 to the costs associated with caring for that person.[2] It's not just the cost. More importantly, this survey found that patients who acquired an infection in hospital were seven times more likely to die in hospital than uninfected patients. But, you might say, it was the seriously ill patients who picked up the infection, so they were more likely to die in the first place. Not so. The researchers came to this conclusion after taking account of the age, sex and degree of illness of each patient.

So which bugs are the biggest threat? A research study in the UK monitored three hospitals in England looking for outbreaks of gastroenteritis in 2002 and 2003. They found a total of 2,154 patients and 1,360 healthcare staff were affected in 227 outbreaks. The most frequent cause of these was Norovirus, a particularly vicious critter that causes diarrhoea and vomiting and which was the agent behind sixty-three per cent of outbreaks. One consequence was that the hospitals lost 5,443 bed-days, equivalent to losing two seven-bed wards for an entire year. When the researchers extrapolated their findings to create an estimate of the total cost of hospital-acquired stomach bugs within the UK, they concluded that the National Health Service lost £115 million in 2002 and 2003.[3] Next comes *Clostridium difficile*, a strain of bacteria that normally lives in our gut, but which often blooms when a person is given antibiotics, and which then causes diarrhoea. The skin-dwelling *Staphylococcus aureus* is another frequent visitor − and we'll see a lot more of it as the chapter goes on.

The commonest sites of healthcare-associated infections are the urinary system, lungs, wounds and the blood stream. The usual routes for the bugs to break in are catheters and tubes put in by medics to drain or supply fluid. While inserting tubes can save lives, they are perfect conduits for disease-causing organisms as they bypass the skin − the body's major means of defence. The longer the tubes are in place, the more likely it is for a problem to arise.

With this sort of information available, it is right to ask hard questions, and one way that politicians and the press often start is by looking beyond the borders and seeing what the situation is in other parts of the world. Sadly, this provides no quick answers. Comparing countries to see which is doing best is normally a waste of time, because each country collects and records its data in different ways. For example, while the rates of particular infections are closely monitored and reported in the UK, it is very difficult to come to any firm conclusions. In the USA, most states do not demand that individual hospitals release their figures on infection rates. This may change slowly, as by 2004 Missouri, Illinois, Pennsylvania and Florida had passed laws requiring hospitals to make infection rates publicly available and in 2005 the majority of states were considering legislation to force this disclosure. In the meantime, best guesses are all you can go on.

A lack of firm knowledge seldom stops accusations of malpractice, and with a background of high numbers of affected patients, it is all too easy to assume that great health benefits and savings are just a quick fix away. Pete Grannis, an assembly member for New York State circulated a memo among his fellow assembly members claiming that, "limiting infections contracted by patients while they are being treated in a hospital can save anywhere between $100 and $200 million dollars in state and local Medicaid expenses per year, and improve healthcare – a true win-win result". He continued, "Requiring hospitals to report [hospital-acquired] infection incidents and setting a date for the release of this information in the hospital report cards... will give them the incentive they need to address this costly and largely avoidable problem."[4]

Talking to infection-control nurses who are at the sharp end of the action in hospitals, there is a fairly uniform view that some hospital-acquired infections (HAIs) are inevitable – a lot can be done to reduce them, but they will never be completely eradicated. This point is strengthened by the fact that HAI rates have remained fairly constant, at around ten per cent, for decades. What's more, over this time the sorts of procedures carried out in hospitals have become vastly more complex, as a result of which people are much more likely to acquire infections, many of them originating from the patients' own flora. The reason why infection rates aren't soaring must therefore be that prevention is in fact getting better. Now this doesn't mean that hospitals should simply sit back and do nothing. But equally, it means that much of the hysterical reporting that suggests every case is a medical mishap is wide of the mark.

The New Bug on the Block

One reason why anxiety levels have risen is the increasing number of bugs that are hard to beat. As we have seen frequently though this book, antibiotics might have given a new sense of security, but antibiotic resistance is bacteria's mechanism of fighting back. Still, this seemed to be only a minor problem because, as bacteria learnt to resist one antibiotic, pharmaceutical companies did a pretty good job of finding new ones that could defeat these tutored bacteria. Or they did well initially. Over the last decade or so, they have hit a bit of a brick wall. It has been difficult to find new ways of thwarting bacteria. In addition, pharmaceutical companies complain that the cost of running the gambit of clinical trials required before a drug can be released has increased dramatically.

The result is that we now have a small range of antibiotics, including methicillin and vancomycin, that can clobber most bacteria, and that are deliberately held back as agents of last resort so that bacteria have never seen them before. Sadly, even these antibiotics have been used to the extent that there are now growing pools of bacteria that can resist the attacks of all known antibiotics.

The headline grabber is MRSA – methicillin-resistant *Staphylococcus aureus*. Most people have this *S. aureus* somewhere on their bodies, most probably millions of them are in the pores of our skin or hiding in our nostrils. They seem to live there quite happily without causing us any harm. Problems start when these colonies get out of control and set up an infection. The result is often a boil, which in the past could have been a killer, but is now soon solved with a course of penicillin or a similar antibiotic. If the bacteria chop up the penicillin instead, then you need to escalate your search for an effective weapon. Ideally, a lab test should sort out which antibiotic stands most chance, but if the answer is that it is resistant to them all, including methicillin, then you are in trouble.

Thankfully, very few strains of bacteria are immune to every antibiotic on the books, because while a bug gains resistance to one it often at the same time loses resistance to another. Consequently, noting that a person has an infection caused by MRSA does not mean that the doctor has just signed his or her death warrant. It does, however, mean that the doctor is going to have to make an intelligent use of a cocktail of antibiotics to beat the foe.

The world's most comprehensive surveillance system looking for MRSA runs in the UK. It was set up in 2001, and researchers soon revealed what they had suspected for some time – this was more than a minor issue. In the year 2001/2002, they recorded 7,249 cases of patients who had MRSA infections in their blood. This number rose to 7,684 by 2003/2004. In a similar manner, the UK's Office for National Statistics records that the number of deaths attributed to MRSA increased from 487 in 1999 to 955 in 2003.

Making sense of these numbers is harder than it might seem at first. After all, the story would appear to be simple – the situation is getting worse. But over this period, the surveillance system has almost certainly been getting better, so it will pick up a higher proportion of cases. It might be that fewer patients are getting sick with this bug, but that we are simply recording more. Either way there are many people who would prefer not to have caught it.

When MRSA first appeared, many – probably most – of the infected people encountered the bacterium for the first time while they were in hospital. It was a hospital-acquired infection – an HAI. But before we throw our hands up in horror and run screaming to our local lawyer, it is worth noting that this doesn't necessarily point to poor care within hospitals. It just makes simple biological sense. Antibiotic-resistant bacteria are going to show up most frequently in places where antibiotics are used most. And it is difficult to beat a hospital for that.

But the situation is now far more complex. The bacterium has been carried out into the community and quite happily lives at low levels on the skin of many people, without causing any problems. Tracking the source of an individual infection is almost impossible because of the way the healthcare system works. The boundaries are not clear – patients who receive healthcare will start by visiting a primary care setting, and then come into hospital for part of that care before going back out into the community and coming back in to the hospital as out-patients. The consequence is that if someone develops an infection it is very difficult to pinpoint where it came from. One way of acknowledging this is to alter the name from Hospital-Acquired Infection (HAI) to Healthcare-Acquired Infection (HCAI).

Even if the disease develops while you are sitting in a hospital bed, it doesn't mean that you picked up the bug in the last few days. When someone goes into hospital they may well be tested to see if they are already carrying bacteria such as MRSA, but this will depend on what they have been admitted for. When swabs are taken from a patient they are normally taken from the nose and any open wounds, as these are the areas where bacteria are most likely to survive. If MRSA isn't found in those areas, it is an indicator that it is not present. However, the organism may be lying dormant anywhere on your body, so the test isn't conclusive. What we do know, though, is that giving people certain antibiotics can clear some bacteria, but the drug makes it easier for others to grow. So you might have a few colonies of MRSA on your skin when you come into hospital. Initially you get a negative result because it wasn't found in your nose and wounds – but when an infection occurs it may be due to organisms which are part of the normal skin flora. In fact this would have happened if you had taken the antibiotics at home. The infection may be an unwanted side effect of the medical treatment, not a consequence of poor hospital care.

C. difficile plays a slightly different game. It is part of the normal gut flora. If you give someone antibiotics, the balance of bacteria in the gut changes and allows the *C. difficile* to proliferate. These can then produce a toxin that causes the diarrhoea – but that is a side effect of the antibiotic, not an error on behalf of a poorly managed hospital. Good management is of course vital. If someone on the ward has explosive diarrhoea the bugs can easily be transferred. So it is then that all the power of good nursing and excellent hygiene needs to be brought to bear. You can't be complacent.

Even so, the complexity doesn't stop there. New strains of MRSA appear to be popping up spontaneously within the community. These are then brought into hospitals hitch-hiking on patients or their visitors. You could easily carry in bacteria when you call in on a friend.

Blame the Cleaner

That said, hospitals should be the places of the greatest concentration of expert knowledge in the area, so it is fair to look at how well they are doing. Setting up league tables to see which hospitals are doing the best jobs of fighting the disease is equally complex. Patients don't sit still, so it's quite possible for someone to catch the bug in one hospital, but for it only to show up after they have been transferred to another.

Before hospital administrators are let off the hook, it's worth noting that no hospital in the Western world is exempt from the problem. In the run-up to a General Election in the UK in May 2005, HCAI suddenly emerged as one of those headline-grabbing stories designed to trip up unsuspecting politicians. The argument soon became focused around the need for better cleaning in hospitals, and the politics of whether private contractors are used for this task.

In a celebrity-driven culture, an issue is only real if some well-known entertainer has it. So with a due flurry of press releases a patients' campaign group convened the "Cleaner Hospitals Summit" a couple of weeks before the election and they almost literally wheeled out Leslie Ash. Leslie had been a highly popular actress in the long running TV sit-com "Men Behaving Badly" and the feminine attraction in a series of TV ads. Married to a former professional football player Lee Chapman, she was part of the jet set. That was until she broke a rib and punctured her lung one evening in April 2004, apparently during a spell of energetic lovemaking, and had a chest drain inserted.[5] To relieve the pain while this drain was inserted, doctors gave an epidural to inject pain-killers directly into her spine. It appears that the epidural also introduced MSSA (methicillin-sensitive *Staphylococcus aureus*), a version of *S. aureus* that is not totally resistant to antibiotics, but resistant enough to cause a significant problem. For Leslie the problem was an abscess that put pressure on her spinal cord and came close to paralysing her. The consequence was that a year later she could only walk with the aid of sticks or crutches. It's easy to trivialise an issue by bringing out a "celeb", but anyone who could remember Leslie bouncing around TV sets a few years ago was bound to be taken aback by the transformation.

No one wants to sit around in a smelly ward, or see discarded dressings lying on the floor. Dirt and dressings will carry bugs. In numerous interviews, Leslie blamed the hospital for her disability, and it was easy for campaigners to use this to garner publicity for their desire to increase the level of cleaning within hospitals. It shows just how easy it is to join the "let's sue 'em" bandwagon. But it is interesting to look at some of the issues to see whether the complaint is justified.

To start with, clean is very different from germ-free. You can sweep all the dirt away, you can also wash a floor with detergent, but you will still leave some bacteria behind. Add some hypochlorite to the solution and you will kill more, but no amount of general cleaning will ever get into every nook and cranny. One of the ways that hospitals get around this is by keeping the environment as clean as possible, but then treating the bed as an especially clean zone. Think hard before sitting on a bed when visiting a patient, because you will carry outside germs into that clean zone.

Full Wards

This emphasis on the cleanliness of the bed space has important implications. It seems that one of the problem areas could be the constant drive for greater efficiency. But efficiency has its limits. Having full beds all the time may be a good way of maximising cash flow, but when are you going to clean them? Studies show that if bed-occupancy goes over seventy per cent, then rates of hospital-acquired infections increase. The reason is simple enough: if beds are full all the time, there is no way a cleaner can make a good job of cleaning a ward.

OK, you can change the sheets between patients, but at some point the bed itself needs cleaning, as does the floor beneath and behind it. You need to empty the wards every now and again so that the whole place can be cleansed – walls, floor, curtains and all. If all the beds in the hospital are full, this just isn't possible, and in a world where things don't quieten down over the weekends, finding the space in a calendar for thorough cleaning can be hard.

A 2004 UK government report complained that hospital occupancy was frequently higher than the eighty-two per cent target that had been set by health policy-makers, and lamented the lack of suitable isolation facilities that could be used for patients who may infect others in the hospital.[6]

The obsession with bed occupancy is an interesting pointer to a critical part of the mindset behind the way hospitals are run. In a management culture driven by targets there is a tendency to concentrate on things that can be counted. Full and empty beds are easy. The "quality" of a person's life or the care they receive are harder to quantify. Maximising output might work well in a factory making cars or washing machines, where you want to ensure that every bay or robot is occupied for the maximum amount of time, but in the less precise world of a hospital, rules need to be more flexible and judgements have to be more subtle.

But in any case, bed occupancy and cleanliness are quite possibly not the major issues. Many surveys show that hospital cleanliness has improved over the first years of the twenty-first century, just at the same time that MRSA has burgeoned. Dirty floors alone can't be the answer. But the cleaner is an easy target because many are poorly educated and are not best equipped to fight back.

Clean Hands

So what are the other possible factors for the increase in HCAI? One clearer culprit is the attitude towards personal hygiene shown by healthcare staff – and by senior medical staff in particular. Obviously hand-washing is at the fore-front of infection control, but my observation is that compliance is poor. I spent twenty-four hours in a UK hospital after suffering an allergic reaction while eating a meal in a pub. As I sat in my bed I spotted on the wall in front of me a dispenser of alcohol-impregnated hand-cleansing gel. The idea is that as hands are the main means of spreading disease, hospital staff and visitors should use it to clean their hands when entering the ward. Did they ever do so? At no point in my stay did I see a consultant go near it, nor did any of the senior nursing staff or junior doctors. I'm not sure whether the cleaner was aware that it existed, nor the man who came around delivering our meals. Now maybe they were using a dispenser that I couldn't see from my bed. Maybe. But it is a comment that you hear repeated by others who have sat and watched. One thing I do know for certain – no one told my visitors that it was there.

There was one measure of success that could bode well for the future. I once saw a group of three nurses come onto the ward. The senior member stood by looking a little awkward while the junior two used the hand-rub gel. They then entered. If the message is getting through to the staff currently being trained, and they keep up the practice once their training is over, then it will only take 40 years before everyone is doing it!

Had I been feeling well, I might have challenged people about their use of this germ-killing system. But I was in there because I wasn't feeling well, and certainly not wanting to do anything that might make me less welcome.

No one came on the ward with mud dripping from their hands. No one, for that matter had any noticeable dirt on his or her hands. But that's not the point. Touch someone with an infection and you will pick up bugs. Touch someone else and, although unseen, you will pass them on.

Antibiotics

The other issue is our over-use of antibiotics. Again, not the fault of the cleaner. If anything, it is rather the fault of medics who should know better. A team of researchers from Belgium compared antibiotic use and antibiotic resistance rates in twenty-six European countries. The study found that the prescription rates of antibiotics in primary care varied greatly, with the highest level being in France and the lowest in the Netherlands. Overall, they found that resistance to antibiotics is more common in southern and eastern Europe than in northern Europe, and then linked this to the higher rates of antibiotic use in the south. One of the authors concluded, "population-based studies are needed to determine the motivation and incentives that lead individuals to use or not to use antibiotics. The ethics of promoting antibiotics in clinical situations in which they are unnecessary should be given serious consideration."

One of the intriguing things is just how well one population of bacteria pass on their learning to another. While MRSA have learned to fight methicillin, VRE is a strain of enterococcus bacteria that have learned to resist vancomycin. They do it by having a set of genes that give them the information needed to build proteins that effectively block the action of each antibiotic. But in research published in 2003, a team of microbiologists at the USA's Centers for Disease Control and Prevention revealed more of the way that the genes collected by *S. aureus* can be traded with those developed by enterococci. This means that in one step a population of *S. aureus* can suddenly become resistant to vancomycin – or a group of enterococci to methicillin.[7]

Other people have started looking for non-antibiotic ways forward. One piece of experimental work suggested that giving a patient good 'ole aspirin reduced the potency of *S. aureus*. It's certainly time to start thinking about looking for these sorts of alternatives.[8]

Deep Cleaning

The need to drive bacteria from wards has created a raft of specialist companies who will show up at a few hours' notice and apply their own patented treatment. While some work by rigorous traditional cleaning with mops and buckets of disinfectant, the more powerful tend to work by sealing the ward and then fumigating it with a chemical that one way or another blasts holes in the outer cell wall of any bacteria or viruses lying around.

A key advantage of the disinfecting chemicals is that bacteria should find them impossible to resist. Bacteria get around antibiotics, because those drugs operate in a sophisticated manner within the machinery of a cell to block specific biochemical pathways. All the bacterium needs to do to resist them is to block the drug or develop a bypass. Chemicals like hydrogen peroxide simply rip the cell apart. It's rough, it's ready and resistance is hopeless.

This may be effective, but is, however, disruptive to hospital life. You need to close and seal a ward, and then pay a sizeable fee to the contractor. It's not something that managers want to do every week.

As a less intrusive approach, other inventors are beginning to place ultra-violet light sources inside the pipes that circulate air through air-conditioning systems. Ultra-violet light treatment has a unique mode of action. Often the UV doesn't kill the target micro-organism, but instead rattles the DNA that holds the bug's genes so that it can't grow or reproduce. If a bacterium cannot proliferate it can't infect and cause disease. Also, an organism that can't reproduce simply dies.

Taking the infective capability out of the air could seem to be one way of making hospitals safer, but the process may be difficult to introduce in an entire hospital. Many do not have forced air supplies and rely on air blowing in and out through windows and doors. On top of this, you would need vast systems to treat the entire volume of air in the building.

There are a couple of rays of hope for this sort of technology. Firstly, it could be used in areas of particular concern, such as isolation units that are used for patients at extreme risk of becoming ill if they encounter any germs. Secondly, it could be used in office environments where air-conditioning is prevalent, and as such might stop people being sent to hospital in the first place!

Doing Your Bit Well

So, if you find yourself in hospital, and want to keep as well as possible, what should you do? First and foremost, keep your hands and body clean. Having a container of moist hand-wipes will enable you to clean your hands. Make sure you take your own toiletries (including soap and a clean flannel) with you – it's going to travel over your body, so you want to know where it has been. Men should take their own razor to avoid any chance of borrowing a razor that may be shared.

As in any environment, always wash your hands after using the toilet. It's not just your own germs you want to get rid of, it's anyone else's that you may have picked up. If you use a commode, ask for a bowl of water to wash your hands, or use a moist hand-wipe afterwards. Wearing something on your feet when walking around the ward, and then kicking these off before getting back into bed will help protect your personal clean zone.

Many people wash their hands after a meal to get the stickiness off, but make sure you do it beforehand – your moist wipes will help here. And keep an eye on the alcohol gels, making sure that, even if they never do it at any other time, staff use them before visiting you. Similarly, never be afraid to point out anything that looks unclean – if the system is working well you should be thanked for your vigilance!

Some Hope

A lot of attention has been focused on hospitals and rightly so. These are places where there is a concentration of highly educated people, and a place of refuge for sick people. They should be natural places where best practice shines out, and if they fall short then everyone should shout. As we have already seen, even if you could clean out all the bacteria (antibiotic-resistant or not) from a hospital one day, it would be re-infected with bugs the next, because patients, visitors, staff and the wind would take the bugs in. The appearance will be of an HCAI – and the temptation will be to blame the system. Actually, the culprit in this case would be basic biology.

A careful analysis of the exact genes carried by the bacteria can give an indication of whether they were carried in from outside, or picked up on the ward, as there are noticeable differences between the groups – but no assessments can say for sure where you first made your acquaintance with the bug.

One hope for the near future comes from developments in gene-scanning technology. Laboratory techniques are coming on-stream that can quickly search through a medical sample looking for bacteria and determining which antibiotics they are resistant to. Rather than the conventional tests that take days to culture the organisms, these can be done in a couple of hours or less. Some claim that this will be reduced to a couple of minutes. As a consequence, doctors will, for example, be able to take a swab from an infected site on a patient, check which organisms are present, and also which antibiotics would have most effect against them. They could then target the infections with appropriate drugs from the start, which should go a long way to reducing the numbers of resistant bacteria, both in hospitals and the community. It would be a great stride towards reducing the chance of getting fatally ill while in hospital.

Reality Check

After the 2005 election in the UK, Patricia Hewitt stepped into the role of Health Secretary and in her first speech annoyed much of the healthcare profession by displaying a cavalier ignorance of the issues. "Not all healthcare-associated infections can be prevented," she said – fine so far, "But we have to do better." Again, not much trouble yet – you can always strive to do better. The trouble came after her next breath. "In my last job as Secretary of State for Trade and Industry, I visited a number of top-class British food production factories. And I now find it absolutely extraordinary that we have tougher laws and higher standards for hygiene in our food factories than we have for hygiene in our hospitals. It is extraordinary and unacceptable. It's not good enough. And together, we have to improve it."[9]

The shock-tactic may make a good headline, but it makes poor common sense. Hospitals and food factories are two totally different places – they are worlds apart. No food manufacturer is going to allow thousands of people, many carrying high levels of nasty bugs, to walk backwards and forwards through their sterile facility. Does she really expect every doctor, nurse, visitor and cleaner – the list could go on – to shower down and change into freshly sterilised clothing and white boots before passing through the doors of their local hospital or entering their GP's clinic? Yes, hospitals need to be run to high standards, but let's work out what a hospital is before making policy.

To have real hope for our hospitals, we need policy-makers who get real. Infection control is a serious issue and everyone who enters a healthcare environment, be they a patient, member of staff or a visitor, needs to admit to his or her personal responsibility. At the same time, we all need to recognise that we are fighting a war against microbes that are great at breaking down our strongest defences, and can easily have a party at our expense when someone's defences are down – it is just part of the way things are.

CHAPTER 15 –
THE RISK OF RECESSION

The battle is ancient. Its origins are lost in the mists of time. But one thing is certain, we, not microbes, are the newcomers. Micro-organisms have a history that is much longer than ours and they are survivors. Human beings have gained an appearance of superiority because we can create tools and deliberately alter environments to suit ourselves. These skills are remarkable and, used well, they stretch us physically and mentally so that we have stepped beyond merely existing and started to enjoy life so that music, art, culture and beauty can all pull at our emotions.

Protozoa, bacteria, viruses and prions don't care. They are blissfully unaware of such complications and are simply devoted to the task of increasing their number. Most have found niches that allow them to exist in ways that benefit the biological community. On occasion, however, their strategy is over-zealous and their mode of action so aggressive that they bite the hand that feeds them. It is against these that we human beings try to target our medical armoury.

The danger for us comes if we ever think that we have won. Micro-organisms will never be beaten, and the last thing we should attempt to do is totally eradicate them. If we succeeded, life on Earth would cease. Most bugs are our friends. We require protozoa to break down decaying material so that it can be recycled. We need bacteria in our guts to help us digest food. Ruminants depend entirely on bacteria to break down the cellulose in grasses so that they can salvage the energy locked up in it. Even viruses play a useful role in moving genes around from place to place, so that other micro-organisms can rapidly adapt to changing circumstances, aiding the evolution of bacteria and higher plants and animals. The problem for us is that sometimes these friendly co-inhabitants of our planet become modified in a way that causes them to do us damage. It's unfortunate for us, and it is not so good for them, because they will either be attacked by our immune systems and get evicted, or they will kill us and, like squatters who have set the house that they have occupied on fire, lose their home.

We will never get rid of infectious disease, because no sooner have we wiped out one offender than another bug will mutate to bring new forms of disease. It appears at the moment that we are only just beginning to understand the scope of infectious diseases. There has been a tendency to restrict our thinking to look only at the obvious outbreaks of disease and think that that is the limit. But now diseases that doctors have for years thought had purely physical causes are being found to have an infective element that either triggers the disease or makes its occurrence more likely.

For decades doctors had treated stomach ulcers by pouring in drugs that radically alter the stomach lining's biochemistry. The rationale was that too much acid in the stomach must have caused the ulcers. Acid is produced by the stomach's lining, so that obvious thing was to give the person drugs that turn off this acid production. Now we know that *Helicobacter pylori* bacteria are the cause of many, if not most, stomach ulcers and doctors attack it using a combination of three different antibiotics. Cancer may also have an infectious accomplice in crime. Cervical cancer is much more likely to strike a woman who is infected with human papilloma virus. Scientists believe that human papilloma virus is also involved in some forms of mouth cancer. In addition, herpes 6 virus might trigger multiple sclerosis.

Statistics show that, year on year, people living in the wealthy West are on average getting fatter. Obesity in children is increasing at an alarming rate. Too much junk food has been blamed, and it is easy to see why as chips and burgers replace apples and pears. But what if obesity was caused by a virus? It's a weird idea, but researchers at the University of Wisconsin Medical School have data suggesting that an infection with adenovirus-36 can induce excessive fat storage. Chickens deliberately infected with the virus put on sixty to seventy-five per cent more fat than uninfected birds, and people who are overweight are much more likely to have antibodies in their blood showing that they have had an infection, than are thin people.

Virtually all children experience a rotavirus infection before starting school and they are the major cause of diarrhoea in young children, accounting for up to fifty per cent of cases admitted to hospital in developed countries. According to the CDC, rotaviruses cause fifty thousand babies to have to go into hospital each year so that they can be treated for dehydration. In developing countries, where there is not the luxury of these facilities, twenty per cent of infant deaths are due to gastroenteritis caused by rotaviruses. Now there is some evidence suggesting that rotaviruses may have a longer-lasting impact – they may also cause diabetes. Working at The Walter and Eliza Hall Institute, Melbourne, Australia, Dr Margo Honeyman suggests that rotavirus epidemics in the past few decades may account for the rising incidence of insulin-dependent diabetes. She also thinks that newly developed vaccines against the virus could reduce the number of children who develop this form of diabetes.

Balancing Risks

A debate on British radio in August 2000 discussed the merits of vaccination[1]. One side argued that vaccination is dangerous, the other that it is safe. As with most of these programmes it was more of a stand-up fight than a meeting of intellects as neither side had any interest in debating, in testing their argument and maybe developing it in the light of evidence presented by their opponents. The pro-vaccination group accused their opponents of hysteria and the anti-vaccination group raised the accusation of conspiracy and cover-up.

There are, I believe, two aspects to this debate. The first involves balancing the risk of your child developing the disease if they are not vaccinated, against the risk of the vaccine itself causing some problem. The fear is that the health authorities are so keen to have a disease-free society that they are less than open in telling people about the potential risks and so try to cover up any evidence of damage. From the health authorities' point of view, mass coverage is essential for vaccination to have any effect. Without the majority of the population accepting the jab the disease-causing agent can still find sufficient hosts and will continue to propagate from person to person.

The second source of heat in the debate then comes from the perceived lack of provision for people who developed disabilities as children. In the UK, parents of these children complain that while there are state-sponsored vaccination campaigns, the social provision of care for people with disabilities is poor.

So can vaccinations damage some children? The chances are that we will probably never know for sure, because the numbers of potentially affected children are small and it is impossible to do an experiment where you confine the children to a closed environment so that you can exclude any other causes of disease. The doctors in favour of vaccination say that a child who becomes disabled after a dose of vaccine would have developed the disability even if it had never been given. It is a coincidence that they received the vaccine just before any symptoms emerged.

Thankfully the debate began to grind to a halt as international trials repeatedly failed to link vaccination with ill-health – but it will take decades for full confidence to return.

The reality that never really emerged in the debate was the spectre of life without vaccinations. It is difficult for those of us living in our relatively healthy enclave in the West to recognise the true threat of infectious disease. It is easy to fall into the false belief that infectious disease is on the retreat and that most peoples around the world live comfortable lives like ours. The truth is that I live as a member of the fortunate minority – the few who enjoy freedom from the fear of a host of diseases. That freedom has been bought first of all by the provision of good social hygiene – sewers and storm-drains – and secondly by vaccines and antibiotics.

Living on the Edge

Our species is facing unprecedented pressures. Population growth has created enormous, sprawling cities. Escalating demands for consumer goods to stoke up the boilers of capitalism require greater and greater exploitation of the natural capital locked up in mines and forests. Exploiting these resources drives people to work in environments that human beings haven't previously encountered. Globalism and rapid, mass international travel stirs the pot of humanity and disease with ever-increasing vigour.

Virologist Japp Goudsmit is anxious: "Monkeys and other animals peacefully harbour many microbes whose potential is as threatening to humans as HIV. The animals and their microbes are content in their equilibrium, but if we destroy the animals or their habitat, the microbes will need a new host. Like HIV, microbes that find a foothold in the human host could use 'viral sex' to adapt, with human disease as the consequence."[2]

Not only do we need to worry about new diseases never before seen in human beings extending their scope and entering our arena for the first time, but we also need to be concerned about the possibility of old diseases gaining new ground. In many quarters we are already witnessing a recession in our health economy, a time when month on month things are getting worse.

"Think about it," challenged Gro Harlem Brundtland, at the conclusion of her contribution to the BBC Reith Lectures, 2000. "Great advances in health care have been made over the past hundred years. Our generation risks going down in history as the one that allowed the hard-won health achievements of the twentieth century to be lost – lost because it decided to ignore the billion and a half people that had been excluded from the health revolution. I use the word 'decided' – because we can't say we failed to act because we didn't know better. The evidence is there – and so are the opportunities. I challenge you to accept this new thinking and act on it."

Past ignorance initially fuelled the pace at which antibiotics went from wonder drugs to potions that can coach superbugs into existence. Past ignorance caused us to rush into developing and implementing vaccines at rates that have quite possibly caused new disease, such as Guillian-Barré syndrome and HIV-AIDS, while knocking out the original target. Current ignorance about the true scale of disease around the world is less forgivable; we know disease exists, but seem unwilling to take it seriously.

"We are in a race against time to bring levels of infectious disease down worldwide before the diseases wear the drugs down first,"[3] says David Heymann, the executive director of the WHO's programme on communicable diseases. In an article on vaccination, journalist Deborah MacKenzie makes the point that, "All the technology in the world won't eliminate an infectious disease if the will isn't there to use it... you can't eradicate measles anywhere if you don't eradicate it everywhere... People in rich countries have forgotten what it is like to lose half their kids to disease."[4]

The WHO 1999 annual report comments that previous generations once prayed for life-saving drugs, interventions and control strategies. "But now that they are available, the world has been slow to put them to wide use. In disease-endemic countries, global efforts have remained embarrassingly modest. Only three per cent of Africa's children have bednets. Effective anti-TB medicines and treatment strategies reach only twenty-five per cent of the world's TB cases... The under-use and misuse of recent health breakthroughs has been catastrophic for people living and working in developing countries."[5]

While wealthy nations focus their attention solely on producing therapies for their own fee-paying people, we play a dangerous game of chicken. The bugs that develop and thrive in poor countries don't need passports and no quarantine system can guarantee to keep them out. While they are nurtured on less than optimum regimens of therapeutic drugs, the bugs learn and develop their skills, so that when they land on wealthy shores they are fit fanatics of destruction.

Resistance is also seen where health workers have exclusively focused on providing drugs for their patients while inadvertently failing to take time to ensure proper diagnosis, prescription and adherence to treatment.

The WHO refers to a "closing window of opportunity" and warns that we need to act quickly. "Before long, we may have forever missed our opportunity to control and eventually eliminate the most dangerous infectious diseases. Indeed, if we fail to make rapid progress during this decade, it may become very difficult and expensive – if not impossible – to do so later. We need to make effective use of the tools we have now. The eradication of smallpox in 1980, for example, happened not a moment too soon. Just a few years' delay and the unforeseen emergence of HIV would have undermined safe smallpox vaccination in populations severely affected by HIV."[6]

Science has a lot of work still to do. Although vaccination continues to be the ultimate weapon against infection and drug resistance, no vaccines exist to shield people from five of the six major infectious killers – respiratory infections, HIV-AIDS, diarrhoeal disease, TB and malaria.

There are glimmers of hope. "Today – despite advances in science and technology – infectious disease poses a more deadly threat to human life than war," warns the WHO. "This year – at the onset of a new millennium – the international community is beginning to show its intent to turn back these microbial invaders through massive efforts against diseases of poverty; diseases which must be defeated now, before they become resistant. When diseases are fought wisely and widely, drug resistance can be controlled and lives saved."[7]

When I started researching for this book, I thought that infectious diseases were merely inconvenient. My impression was that they should never be a serious threat to anyone who looks after their health. I was under the impression that modern medicine had the problem under control. How could I have made this mistake?

Part of the blame needs to be placed on the media, and being a science journalist I have to look to see if some of it lies at my feet. News is in danger of becoming an industry that provides the information we want to hear, rather that the facts we need to know. Concorde crashed while taking off from a Paris airport and the world's media rushed to cover the story, which included the tragic loss of 109 lives. An explosion on the *Kursk*, a Russian submarine, causes it to sink with the loss of 118 lives. Again it is tragic and it is easy to focus on single events that cause many deaths.

These were newsworthy events. But the sad reality is that the numbers of people involved are desperately small compared with the statistics for almost any infectious disease. The problem is that death from disease is no longer newsworthy simply because of the monotonous regularity with which people die. Being out of the news, it is easy for us to rush by as if it is not an issue. Occasionally the arrival of a new bug, such as nvCDJ, does make the headlines. The reason is that it is new and it is a good scare story. All the same, few people point out that you are more likely to die as a result of 'flu, or to be incapacitated because of a stomach ulcer or food poisoning caused by ignoring basic hygiene.

The buzzword of the twenty-first century is globalism. Governments and industries are trying to work out what it is to live and work in a world where transport and information technology link everyone in a global village. Bugs have always been aware of just how small the world is and have made good use of its high degree of interconnectedness to propagate their presence. As wealthy nations seek to exploit this global marketplace, they need to adopt an attitude of care and responsibility that does all it can to move medical technology into these areas with the same enthusiasm that they move industrial technology.

They could do this from one of two motives. The first would be from the fear that unless they prevent the build-up of disease in these "far-away" lands, then the health of the home nations is at risk. And that is undoubtedly true. On the other hand, they could be motivated by a nobler cause that recognises their ability to help fellow human beings and seek to do everything to bring good health to as many people as possible. It would be exciting to seek the moral high ground and adopt a principle of altruism in the way that we seek to arrest disease, and give people the freedom of good health.

Infectious diseases are here to stay. Our task is to give them as little room for manoeuvre as possible lest they develop their skills and become pandemic-causing killer germs.

NOTES

Chapter One: CONTEMPORARY COMPLACENCY

1 1996 WHO Annual Report.
2 "Removing Obstacles to Healthy Development" (1999) WHO.
3 *Journal of the American Medical Association* (1996) 275: pp.189–193.
4 T.B. Macaulay. *The History of England from the Accession of James II*, Vol IV.
5 Baron J. *Life of Edward Jenner*. London: H Colburn; 1827 (v 1), 1838 (v 2).
6 "The management and control of hospital-acquired infection in acute NHS trusts in England". National Audit Office. 14 Feb 2000. p. 17.
7 Hospital infections cost NHS £1bn a year. Reported in: *The Guardian* January 19, 2000.
8 *The Path to Least Resistance* – Chapter 3. "A report of the Standing Medical Advisory Committee – Sub-Group on Antimicrobial Resistance" (1998). Department of Health, London.
9 *The Path to Least Resistance* p.14.
10 McCormick JB (1998) "Epidemiology of emerging/re-emerging antimicrobial-resistant bacterial pathogens". *Current Opinion in Microbiology* 1: pp.125–129.

Chapter Two: LESSONS FROM HISTORY

1 Galimand M, Guiyoule A, Gerbaud G, Rasoamanana B, Chanteau S, Carniel E and Courvalin P (1997) "Multidrug resistance in *Yersinia pestis* mediated by a transferable plasmid". *New England Journal of Medicine* 337: pp.677–680.
2 Dennis D & Hughes J (1997) "Multidrug Resistance in Plague". *New England Journal of Medicine* 337: pp.702–704.
3 Jenner E. "The origin of the vaccine inoculation". London: Printed for the author by DN Shury; 1801.
4. Fine PE, Carnerio IA (1999) "Transmissibility and persistence of oral polio vaccine viruses: implications for the global poliomyelitis eradication initiative." *AMJ Epicemiol* 150: pp.1000–1021.
5 Mackenzie D (2000) "Down but not out." *New Scientist* February 5, 2000. pp.20–21.
6 Charatran F. (2003) "US doctors investigate more than 50 possible cases of monkeypox." *British Medical Journal* 326: p. 1350.
7 "As many as 33 Monkeypox cases diagnosed now." Associated Press. June 6, 2003.
8 So far, 85 monkeypox cases in US outbreak: CDC. Reuters. June 19, 2003.
9 "Multistate outbreak of monkeypox - Illinois, Indiana and Wisconsin, 2003." *MMWR Weekly* June 13, 2003.
10 "Update: Multistate outbreak of monkeypox - Illinois, Indiana, Kansas, Missouri, Ohio and Wisconsin, 2003." *MMWR Weekly* June 20, 2003.
11 Update: Multistate outbreak of monkeypox - Illinois, Indiana, Kansas, Missouri, Ohio and Wisconsin. *MMWR Weekly* July 11, 2003.
12 Stern, A. "U.S. urges smallpox vaccine for monkeypox exposure." Reuters. 11 June, 2003
13 "CDC recommends smallpox vaccination to protect persons exposed to Monkeypox." Centers for Disease Control. June 11, 2003

Chapter Three: BACTERIA AND ANTIBIOTICS

1   Papperheimer AM & Murphy JR (1983) "Studies on the molecular epidemiology of diphtheria". *Lancet* 2: pp. 923–926.
2   Waksman S.A. (1958) "The microbiology of soil and the antibiotics". In: *The Impact of the Antibiotics on Medicine and Society.* (Ed: Galdston I) International Universities Press, Inc. New York, p.3.
3   "Anti-tuberculosis drug resistance in the world". The WHO/IUATLD Global Project on Anti-tuberculosis drug resistance surveillance. 1997.

Chapter Four: ENGINEERING ARMAGEDDON

1   Derbes VJ (1966) "De Mussis and the Great Plague of 1348. A forgotten episode of bacteriological warfare." *Journal of the American Medical Association* 196: 59–62.
2   Quoted in *The Problem of Chemical and Biological Warfare*, Volume 1, SIPRI, Almqvist and Wiksell, Stockholm, 1971, p. 215.
3   In a speech on October 27, 1999 at the Weill Medical College at Cornell University. www.news.cornell.edu
4   Reported in *New Scientist* September 1, 2001, p. 6
5   Quoted in: *Britain battles Chemical, Biological Horrors of War* by Paul Majendie. Reuters, July 31, 1994.
6   A rough translation of the verse from the Bible, Matthew 26:51 "for all who draw the sword will die by the sword."
7   Reported in *New Scientist* October 6, 2001, p. 7
8   "PrimeTime" Febuary 25, 1998.
9   Departments of the Army, Navy and Air Force, *NATO Handbook on the Medical Aspects of NDC Defensive Operations* (Washington, DC, February1996).
10 Dixon TC, Meselson M, Guillemin J & Hanna PC (1999) Anthrax. The New England Journal of Medicine 341: 815–826.
11 Mourez M, Kane RS, Mogridge J, Deschatelets P, Sellman BR, Whitesides GM & Collier RJ (2001) "Designing a polyvalent inhibitor of anthrax toxin." *Nature Biotechnology* 19: 958–961.
12 Henderson DA (1998) Bioterrorism as a public health threat. *Emerging infectious disease* 4: 488
13 Henderson DA (1999) The looming threat of bioterrorism. *Science* 283, 1279–1299.
14 Speaking on "PrimeTime" – February 25, 1998.
15 Miller J & Broad WJ (1998) "Iranians, bioweapons in mind, lure needy ex-Soviet scientists." *New York Times* December 8, 1998, p. A1.
16 U.S. Senate Permanent Subcommittee on Investigations (Minority Staff), Global Proliferation of Weapons of Mass Destruction, a Case Study on the Aum Shinrikyo: Hearing before the Permanent Subcommittee on Investigations, 104th Congress, 1st Sess., October 31, 1995, p. 44.
17 Paul Mann, Mass Weapons Threat Deepens Worldwide. *Aviation Week and Space Technology* June 17, 1996, p. 61.
18 Quoted in the *New York Times* September 30, 2001 "Some see U.S. as vulnerable to Germ Attack."
19 MacLehose L, Brand H, Camaroni I, Fulop N, Gill ON, Reintjes R; Schaefer O, McKee M & Weinberg J. (2001) "Communicable disease outbreaks involving more than one country: systems approach to evaluating the response." *British Medical Journal* 323: 861–863.
20 Speaking to the US Senate Foreign Relations Committee.

Chapter Five: ANTIBIOTIC RESISTANCE

1   "Overcoming Antimicrobial Resistance" – World Health Report on Infectious Disease 2000. Epilogue.
2   Reported in: *New York Times* p. 21, June 26, 1945.
3   Gerard Didier Erasmus (c.1465–1536)
4   Galimand M, Guiyoule A, Gerbaud G, Rasoamanana B, Chanteau S, Carniel E and Courvalin P (1997) "Multidrug resistance in *Yersinia pestis* mediated by a transferable plasmid". *New England Journal of Medicine* 337: pp. 677–680.
5   Lehmann J (1946) "Para-aminosalicyclic acid in the treatment of tuberculosis". *The Lancet* Volume I: pp. 15–16.
6   "Anti-tuberculosis drug resistance in the world" (1997) World Health Organisation.
7   Sledzik Ps & Bellantoni N (1994) "Brief communication: bioarcheological and biocultural evidence for the New England vampire folk belief". *Am J Phys Anthropol* 94 (2): pp. 269–274, 1994.
8   McMurry LM, Oethinger M & Levy SB (1998) "Triclosan targets lipid synthesis". *Nature* 394: 531–532.
9   British Veterinary Assocations (2000) "Guidelines on the prudent use of antimicrobials". BVA Publications. p. 1.
10 Reported in *Infection Disease News* – April 1999. www.slackinc.com.
11 DANMAP 99 – "Consumption of antimicrobial agents and occurrence of antimicrobial resistance in bacteria from food animals, food and humans in Denmark". Published by Danish Veterinary laboratory, Bülowsvej 27, DK 1790 Copenhagen V, Denmark.
12 First reported in May 2000 in *BioMedNet Conference Reporter*. news.bmn.com.
13 Advisory Committee on the Microbial Safety of Food. Microbial Antibiotic Resistance in Relation to Food Safety. Department of Health. HMSO, London. para 8.pp. 30–8.31
14 Levy, Stuart (1992) *The Antibiotic Paradox*. p.152.
15 Quoted in *Sunday Times* colour supplement. February 4, 2000.
16 ibid.

Chapter Six: BIRD FLU: A VAGRANT VIRUS

1   Quoted in Laurie Garrett's book, *The Coming Plague*. p.157.
2   Centers for Disease Control, "Influenza Vaccine – Supplemental Statement," *Morbidity and Mortality Weekly Report* 25 (1976): pp. 221–227.
3   *Canadian Medical Association Journal* (1997) 157: pp. 1573–1574.
4   "On a wing and a prayer". *Nature* (2005) 435 p.385.
    Deborah Mackenzie, 'Bird 'Flu Outbreak Started a Year Ago', *New Scientist January 31, 2004*.
5   *New Scientist* January 31, 2004
6   Kigson N. (2005) "Sit up and take notice about avian flu." *British Medical Journal* 330: p. 1087.
7   Tamblyn SE. (1997) "Amantadine use in influenza outbreaks in long-term care facilities." *Canadian Medical Association Journal* 157: pp. 1573–1574.

Chapter Seven: SARS – OVERDUE PANDEMIC OR ALARMIST PANIC?

1   "Acute respiratory syndrome, China." *Weekly epidemiological record* 2003; 78(7): 41.
2   "Acute respiratory syndrome, China – update." *Weekly epidemiological record*. 2003;78(9):57.
3   Audra Ang, "Earliest known SARS case anonymous – and likely to stay that way.", *Associated Press*, April 12, 2003.

4   Audra Ang, *Associated Press*, April 12, 2003.
5   "Severe Acute Respiratory Syndrome (SARS) – multi-country outbreak – update 24." World Health Organisation. April 8, 2003.
6   Oransky I. Carlo Urbani (2003) *Lancet* 361: p. 1481.
7   Chan-Yeung M & YuWC. (2003) "Outbreak of severe acute respiratory syndrome in Hong Kong Special Administrative Region: case report." *British Medical Journal* 326: p. 850.
8   Benitez MA.(2003) "Hong Kong health chief falls ill with suspected SARS virus." *Lancet* 361; p. 1106.
9   SARS suspected as Hong Kong medical head falls ill. CBC Canada. March 24, 2003.
10 Benitez MA. (2003) "Hong Kong health chief falls ill with suspected SARS virus." *Lancet* 361; p. 1106.
11 Kondro W. (2003) "SARS virus claims its third victim in Canada." *Lancet* 361: p. 1106.
12 Lindsey H. (2003) "AACR cancels annual meeting because of SARS." *The Lancet Oncology* 4: p. 266.
13 Gonzales SO. "SARS: Who began it all when and where?" *The Nation*. April 11, 2003.
14 Smith R. (2003) "After war, plague." *British Medical Journal* 326: p. 1.
15 Chan-Yeung M & Yu WC.(2003) "Outbreak of severe acute respiratory syndrome in Hong Kong Special Administrative Region: case report." *British Medical Journal* 326: p. 850.
16 Tomlinson B & Cockram C. (2003) "SARS: experience at Prince of Wales Hospital, Hong Kong." *Lancet* 361: pp 1486–1487.
17 Rainer TH, et al.(2003) "Evaluation of WHO criteria for identifying patients with severe acute respiratory syndrome out of hospital: prospective observational study." *British Medical Journal* 326: pp 1354–1358.
18 Tomlinson B & Cockram C. (2003) "SARS: experience at Prince of Wales Hospital, Hong Kong." *Lancet* 361: pp 1486–1487.
19 Hesketh T. (2003) "China in the grip of SARS." *British Medical Journal* 326 (May 17): pp 1095
20 Kondro W. (2003) "Canada fury at WHO ban." *Lancet* 361: p. 1525.
21 Spurgeon D. (2003) "Canada reports more than 300 suspected cases of SARS." *British Medical Journal* 326: p. 897.
22 Parry J. (2003) "WHO warns that death rate from SARS could reach 10%." *British Medical Journal* 326: p. 999.
23 "Update: Severe acute respiratory syndrome – United States, June 18, 2003". *Morbidity and Mortality Weekly Review* 2003; 52(24); p. 570.
24 Spurgeon D. (2003) "Toronto succumbs to SARS a second time." *British Medical Journal* 326: p. 1162
25 Market report: Air filters. *Filtration Industry Analyst*. May 2003.
26 Peiris JSM et al. (2003) "Coronavirus as a possible cause of severe acute respiratory syndrome." *Lancet* 361: pp 1319–1325.
27 Kamps & Hoffmann. SARSreference.com. 05/2003. p20.
28 Rainer T. (2003) "Evaluation of WHO criteria for identifying patients with severe acute respiratory syndrome out of hospital: prospective observational study." *British Medical Journal* 326: pp 1354–1358.
29 Wong RSM *et al.* (2003) "Haematological manifestations in patients with severe acute respiratory syndrome: retrospective analysis." *British Medical Journal* 326: pp 1358–1362.
30 Ding Y *et al.* (2003) "The clinical pathology of severe acute respiratory syndrome (SARS): a report from China." *Journal of Pathology* 200: pp.282–289.
31 Ding Y et al. (2004) "Organ distribution of severe acute respiratory syndrome (SARS)

associated coronavirus (SARS-CoV) in SARS patients: implications for pathogenesis and virus transmission pathways." *Journal of Pathology* 203; pp 622–630.

32 Hamming I, Timens W, Bulthuis MLC, Lely AT, Navis GJ and Van Goor H. (2004) "Tissue distribution of ACE2 protein, the functional receptor for SARS Coronavirus. A first step in understanding SARS pathogenesis." *Journal of Pathology* 203(2): pp. 631–637.

Chapter Eight: AIDS

1 Levy JA, Hoffman AD, Kramer SM, Landis JA, Shimabukuro JM, Oshiro LS. (1984) "Isolation of lymphocytopathic retroviruses from San Francisco patients with AIDS". *Science* 225: pp. 840–842.

2 Gallo RC, Sarin PS, Gelmann EP, Robert-Guroff M, Richardson E, Kalyanaraman VS, Mann D, Sidhu GD, Stahl RE, Zolla-Pazner S, Leibowitch J, Popovic M. (1983) "Isolation of human T-cell leukemia virus in acquired immune deficiency syndrome (AIDS)". *Science* 220: 4599 pp. 865–867.

3 Barré-Sinoussi F, Chermann JC, Rey F, Nugeyre MT, Chamaret S, Gruest J, Dauguet C, Axler-Blin C, Vézinet-Brun F, Rouzioux C, Rozenbaum W, Montagnier L (1983) "Isolation of a T-lymphotropic retrovirus from a patient at risk for acquired immune deficiency syndrome (AIDS)". *Science* 220: 4599 pp. 868–871.

4 Investigation of the institutional response to the HIV blood test patent dispute and related matters. OS US House of Representatives; Subcommittee on Oversight and Investigations Committee on Energy and Commerce. DT9501.

5 Shilts, R (1987) *And The Band Played On.* St Martin's Press: New York. p.138.

6 Carey RF, Herman WA, Retta SM, Rinaldi JE, Herman BA, Athey TW (1992) "Effectiveness of latex condoms as a barrier to human immunodeficiency virus-sized particles under conditions of simulated use", *Sex Transm Dis* 19(4): pp. 230–234.

7 Centers for Disease Control and Prevention, *HIV/AIDS Prevention Training Bulletin* January 28, 1993.

8 Hooper E, (2000) *The River.* p.11.

9 Gao F, Bailes E, Robertson DL, Chen Y, Rodenburg CM, Michael SF, Cummins LB, Arthur LO, Peeters M, Shaw GM, Sharp PM, Hahn BH. (1999) "Origin of HIV-1 in the chimpanzee *Pan troglodytes troglodytes*". *Nature* 397: pp. 436–441.

10 Quoted in *The Biochemist.* December 1998. p. 20.

11 Vocero-Akbani AM, Heyden NV, Lissy NA, Ratner L, Dowdy SF. (1999) "Killing HIV-infected cells by transduction with an HIV protease-activated caspase-3 protein". *Nature Medicine* 5: pp. 29–33.

12 Stephenson J (2000) "Apocalypse Now: HIV/AIDS in Africa exceeds the experts' worst predictions". *Journal of the American Medical Association* 284: p.556.

Chapter Nine: . . . AND THEN YOU DISSOLVE

1 WHO Fact Sheet No 117. "Dengue and dengue haemorrhagic fever". Revised 1998.

Chapter Ten: THE VIRAL GOOD GUYS

1 English mathemetician Augustus De Morgan (1806–1871): *A Budget of Paradoxes,* p. 377.

2 "L'action bacericide des Eaux de la Jumma et du Gange sur le vibrion du cholera." Hankin, E.H. (1896). *Ann. de l'Inst. Pasteur* 10: p. 511

3 d'Hérelle FH (1922) in *The Bacteriophage: Its Role in Immunity,*. trans. Smith GH (Williams & Wilkins, Baltimore).

4 Eaton and Bayne-Jones (1931) "Bacteriophage Therapy". *Journal of the American Medical Association* 103: pp. 1769–1776; pp. 1847–1853; pp. 1934–1939.

5   BBC "Horizon" – "The virus that cures".
6   Soothill JS (1994) "Bacteriophage prevents destruction of skin grafts by *Pseudomonas aeruginosa*". *Burns*; 20: pp. 209–211.
7   Merril CR, Biswas B, Carlton R, Jensen NC, Creed GJ, Zullo S, Adhya S. (1996) "Long-circulating bacteriophage as antibacterial agents". *Proc Natl Acad Sci* 93: pp. 3188–3192.
8   Slopek S, Weber-Dabrowska B, Dabrowski M, Kucharewicz-Krukowska A. (1986) "Results of bacteriophage treatment of suppurative bacterial infections in the years 1981–1986". *Arch Immunol Ther Exp (Warsz)* 35: pp. 569–583.

Chapter Eleven: PR IS FOR PRIONS

1   Prusiner, SB (1995) "The prion diseases". *Scientific American*. 272: pp. 48–57.
2   Described in Gadjusek DC (1996) "Kuru in the New Guinea field journals 1957–1962". Grand Street; 12:pp. 6–33.
3   Lindenbaum S (1979) *Kuru Sorcery*. Mountain View, Ca, Mayfield Publishing Company.
4   http://www.nobel.se/medicine/laureates/1997/prusiner-autobio.html
5   Latarjet R, Muel B, Haig DA, Clarke MC & Alper T (1976) *Nature* 277: pp. 1341–1343.
6   Prusiner S (1982) "Novel proteinaceous infectious particles cause scrapie". *Science* 216: pp. 136–144.
7   Will RG, Ironside JW, Zeidler M, Cousens SN, Estiberio K, Alperovitch A, Poser S, Pocchiari M, Hofman A & Smith PG. (1996) "A new variant of Creutzfeldt-Jakob disease in the UK". *Lancet* 347: pp. 921–925.
8   Collinge JRM. (1996) "A new variant of prion disease". *Lancet* 347: pp. 916–917.
9   For regularly updated figures you can visit www.cjd.ed.ac.uk/figures.htm
10 Andrews NJ, Farrington CP, Cousens SN, Smith PG, Ward H, Knight RSG, Ironside JW & Will RG (2000) "The incidence of variant Creutzfeldt-Jakob disease in the UK". *The Lancet* 356: pp. 481–482.
11 Ghani AC, Ferguson NM, Donnelly CA & Anderson RM (2000) "Predicted vCJD mortality in Great Britain". *Nature* 404: pp. 583–584.
12 Reported in *The Sunday Times* July 22, 2000
13 www.cdc.gov/ncidod/dvrd/vcjd/epidemiology.htm. You can follow these test results as they come in at www.aphis.usda.gov/lpa/issues/bse_testing/test_results.html

Chapter Twelve: THE MIGHTY MOSQUITO

1   From: Ronald Ross (1923) *Memoirs With a Full Account of the Great Malaria Problem & Its Solution*.
2   Reported in: "Overcoming Antimicrobial Resistance", World Health Report on Infectious Diseases 2000. Chapter 4.
3   In: *Bailliere's Clinical Infectious Diseses – Malaria*. Baillière Tindal, London (1995). Chapter 1.
4   "Outbreak of West Nile-like viral encephalitis – New York, 1999". *Morbidity and Mortality Weekly Report* October 1, 1999; 48(38): pp. 845–849.
5   Reported in the *New York Times* August 8, 2000. "Clues to an Alien Virus" by Andrew Revkin.
6   Reported in *Environmental News Network*. www.enn.com/news.
7   Reported in the *New York Times* August 8, 2000. "Clues to an Alien Virus" by Andrew Revkin.
8   Reported in *New Scientist* August 12, 2000. p 11.
9   Reported in the *New York Times* August 8, 2000. "Clues to an Alien Virus" by Andrew Revkin.
10 Reported in *BioMedNet Conference Reporter*. news.bmn.com

Chapter Thirteen: FOOT-AND-MOUTH

1   "Unity over foot and mouth jabs." *The Daily Telegraph* September 8, 2001

Chapter Fourteen: HEALTHCARE-ACQUIRED INFECTIONS

1   Getting ahead of the curve – a strategy for infection diseases (including other aspects of health protection), Department of Health. 2002
2   Plowman R *et al*. (1999) Socio-economic burden of hospital-acquired infection. Central Public Health Laboratory. London School of Hygiene & Tropical Medicine.
3   Lopman BA et al. (2004) "Epidemiology and cost of nosocomial gastroenteritis, Avon, England, 2002–2003." *Emerging infectious diseases* 10(10): pp 1827–1834.
4   www.consumersunion.org/campaigns/pete_grannis_memorandum.pdf.
5   http://news.bbc.co.uk/1/hi/uk/3923779.stm.
6   Improving patient care by reducing the risk of hospital-acquired infection: a progress report. 12 July 2004.
7   Weigel L *et al*. (2003) "Genetic analysis of a high level vancomycin resistant isolate of *Staphylococcus aureus.* "*Science* 302: pp 1569–1571.
8   Kupferwasser L.I. *et al*. (2003) "Salicylic acid attenuates virulence in endovascular infections by targeting global regulatory pathways in *Staphylococcus aureus*." *Journal of Clinical Investigation* 112: pp 222–233.
9   Speech by Rt Hon Patricia Hewitt MP, Secretary of State for Health, May 13, 2005: Speech to HR in the NHS Conference.

Chapter Fifteen: THE RISK OF RECESSION

1   BBC Radio 4. "MidWeek" August 9, 2000.
2   Goudsmit, Japp. (1997) *Viral sex – the nature of AIDS*. OUP, Oxford and New York. p. XIX.
3   *Guardian Weekly* June 15–21, 2000.
4   *New Scientist* January 29, 2000. p. 43.
5   "Overcoming Antimicrobial Resistance" – World Health Report on Infectious Disease 2000. Preface.
6   "Overcoming Antimicrobial Resistance" – World Health Report on Infectious Disease 2000. Preface.
7   *ibid*

BIBLIOGRAPHY

Barnaby, Wendy. The Plague Makers. Vision paperbacks, London. 1999.

Barry GM. *The Great Influenza: The Epic Story of the Deadliest Plague in History*. Penguin, New York. 2005.

Chaitow, Leon. The Antibiotic Crisis. HarperCollins, London. 1998.

Davis M. *The Monster at Our Door: The Global Threat of Avian Flu*. The New Press, New York. 2005.

Garrett, Laurie. *The Coming Plague*. Penguin, New York. 1995.

Goudsmit, Japp. *Viral Sex – The Nature of AIDS*. OUP, Oxford and New York. 1997.

Harrison, Polly F. and Lederberg, Joshua, Eds. *Antimicrobial Resistance: Issues and Opinions*. National Academy Press, Washington DC. 1998.

Hooper, Edward. *The River – A Journey Back to the Source of HIV And AIDS*, Penguin, London. 2000.

Levy, Jay. *HIV And The Pathogenesis of AIDS*. American Society for Microbiology, Washington DC. 1998.

Levy, Stuart. *The Antibiotic Paradox – How Miracle Drugs Are Destroying The Miracle*. Plenum Press, New York and London. 1992.

McKeganey, Neil and Barnard, Marina. *AIDS, Drugs and Sexual Risk – Lives In The Balance*. OUP, Buckingham and Philadelphia. 1992.

Preston, Richard. *The Hot Zone*. Random House, New York. 1994.

Wainwright, Milton. *Miracle Cure – The Story of Antibiotics*. Basil Blackwell, Oxford. 1990.

Walters MJ. *Six Modern Plagues: And How We Are Causing Them*. Island Press, Washington, D.C. 2004.

ACKNOWLEDGMENTS

Writing this book was made all the more enjoyable by the help and encouragement of Rachel Quinlan, Yom Lumbers, Mandy Little, Sarah Larter and Adèle Moore. Thanks.

INDEX

PICTURE CREDITS

The publishers would like to thank the following sources for their kind permission to reproduce the pictures in this book:

Plate 1:	Science Photo Library/Eye of Science
Plate 2:	Corbis/Bettman
Plate 3:	Science Photo library/A. Gragera, Latin Stock
Plate 4 – 6:	Hulton Getty
Plate 7:	Hulton Getty/J.A. Hampton
Plate 8:	Corbis/Bettman
Plate 9:	Science Photo Library/Dr. Tony Brain
Plate 10:	AKG London
Plate 11:	The Art Archive/Musee des Beaux Arts, Marseilles
Plate 12:	Hulton Getty/Alan Band Agency
Plate 13:	Advertising Archives
Plate 14:	Science Photo Library/Biozentrum, University of Basel
Plate 15:	Hulton Getty
Plate 16 & 17:	Rex Features/SIPA Press
Plate 18:	Associated Press/Santiago Llanquia
Plate 19 & 20:	Pete Moore

Every effort has been made to acknowledge correctly and contact the source and/copyright holder of each picture, and Carlton Books Limited apologises for any unintentional errors or omissions. Please address all corrections to Citadel Press.

GREAT BOOKS,
GREAT SAVINGS!

When You Visit Our Website:
www.kensingtonbooks.com
You Can Save 30% Off The Retail Price
Of Any Book You Purchase!

- **All Your Favorite Kensington Authors**
- **New Releases & Timeless Classics**
- **Overnight Shipping Available**
- **All Major Credit Cards Accepted**

Visit Us Today To Start Saving!
www.kensingtonbooks.com

All Orders Are Subject To Availability.
Shipping and Handling Charges Apply.